STAND UP TO SLIM DOWN

A 9-Week Program
of Mind-Body Transformation

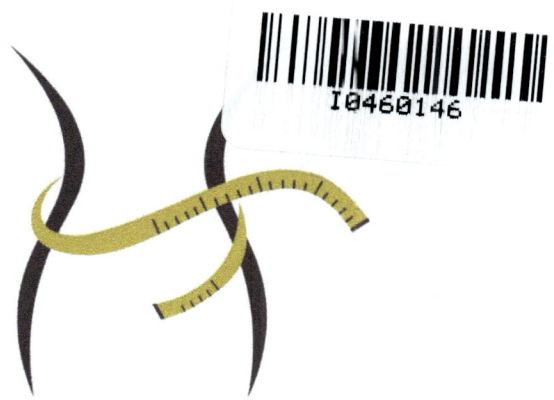

Turn Emotional Weight to Physical Wellness
with Hypnosis

LIZA BOUBARI

ISBN 979-8-9925681-1-0 (print)

ISBN 979-8-9925681-2-7 (ePub)

Library of Congress Control Number: 2025906703

Second Edition

Published by HealWithin, Inc.
330 Arden Ave Suite 130
Glendale CA 91203
www.healwithin.com

DEDICATION

To every woman who has carried not only the weight on her body but the unspoken weight of her emotions—this book is for you.

May it remind you that your worth has never been measured in pounds, but in the power of your presence, the depth of your heart, and the courage it takes to begin again.

This journey isn't just about slimming down. It's about shedding old stories you still carry, releasing shame, and standing up for your health, your happiness, and your voice.

To the women who are learning to listen to their bodies, nourish their needs, and love themselves fully—
May you **Evoke** what was, **Embrace** what is, and **Evolve** into the vibrant, free, and empowered woman you are becoming.

And to my cherished grandmother and mother—
Your quiet strength, love for healing from the inside out, and example of living with grace inspire every step of my work.

You Matter.
With love and honor,

Liza

Table of Contents

INTRODUCTION

Transformation begins with a single step, and you have already taken it by picking up this book. This is no accident—you are here for a reason. You are ready to release the emotional burdens and patterns that have kept you stuck and step into a life of health, balance, and confidence.

Spiritual awakening is when you realize that what's been weighing you down isn't just physical; it's emotional, mental, and even spiritual. The good news is that the same universal energy that created you can also heal you. By aligning with this energy, you can shed pounds and limiting beliefs and habits that no longer serve you.

This book is your guide to releasing what's been eating at you, so you can stand tall, live lighter, and embrace the vibrant, joyful life you deserve.

Lovingly,

Liza

"We must live in the joy of promise and recall that every human being has a unique perception and method of programming their world until they decide to amend it." ~ Liza

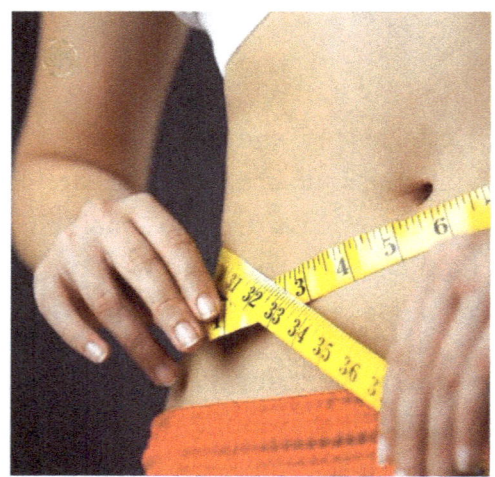

Why Stand Up to Slim Down?

This book is a labor of love, created specifically for women like you—women ready to reclaim their confidence, embrace their bodies, and transform their lives from the inside out.

Over the years, I've witnessed a common thread among my clients: the challenges they face with weight are rarely just about food. Instead, these challenges are deeply rooted in emotions, beliefs, and experiences that shape their self-worth and body image.

For many of us, the journey to a healthier, slimmer self-starts not with diet plans or workout routines but with the courage to **stand up** for who we are. It's about learning to show up authentically, speak up for our needs, and believe that we are worthy of the change we desire.

Stand Up to Slim Down is more than a book—it's a guide to reconnecting with your body and mind, letting go of the weight of past hurts, and stepping into a healthier, more empowered version of yourself. This program is designed to help you peel back the layers of trauma, self-doubt, and limiting beliefs that have held you back. It's about healing from what's been eating at you emotionally, as much as what you've been eating physically.

The 3E Method: Evoke, Embrace, Evolve

The principles of this book are rooted in my signature Boubari 3E Method:

- **Evoke – What Was:** Acknowledge your history, patterns, and experiences with food, your body, and self-perception.

- **Embrace – What Is:** Accept and honor yourself as you are today, without judgment, creating space for clarity and peace.

- **Evolve – To What Will Be:** Visualize and step into the body and life you truly desire, using tools to guide and sustain your transformation.

This method bridges the gap between your conscious mind and your subconscious feelings, offering a holistic approach to change.

Why Now?

If you've ever felt stuck, trying every diet or fitness plan only to end up back where you started, it's not because you lack willpower. It's because real change requires addressing your journey's emotional and mental aspects, not just the physical.

The Stand Up to Slim Down is a 9-week program is your invitation to take control of your health and well-being, not through restrictive measures, but by unlocking the potential already within you. Together, we will explore:

- How your thoughts and emotions impact your body.

- What's been weighing you down emotionally?

- How to release self-sabotaging habits and embrace empowering beliefs.

What You'll Gain

By committing to this journey, you will:

- Heal emotional wounds tied to food and self-image.

- Transform fear and anxiety into self-confidence and clarity.

- Cultivate gratitude and self-love as the foundation for your transformation.

- Discover a sustainable path to living lighter—both physically and emotionally.

A Personal Invitation

You have the power to change, and this book is here to remind you of that. *Stand Up to Slim Down* is not just about losing weight—it's about shedding the layers of what no longer serves you so you can step boldly into the life you've envisioned.

Together, let's embark on this transformative journey. Say yes to yourself and remember: You are worth it.

"To find yourself, think for yourself." ~ Socrates

Let's Stand Up to Slim Down

Everyone desires to improve some aspect of their life—whether it's dropping a few pounds, adopting healthier habits, or embracing a more positive mindset. Often, the root of these desires lies in changing old patterns that no longer serve us. Habits shape who we are, and when we become aware of those holding us back from our goals, it becomes clear that change is necessary.

Yet, many goals we set lack authenticity or a true connection to our mind and body. We tell ourselves, "Life gets in the way," or "It's impossible," only to feel defeated and believe in limits that don't exist. We may explore new ideas or form plans, but without clarity or commitment, these efforts fail to take root.

Some visualize their desired transformation but unknowingly sabotage their efforts by giving up too soon. Is it possible that you, too, have remained in a place of discomfort simply because it feels familiar?

If you struggle to gain weight or find yourself starving for thinness, the craving you feel likely runs deeper than food. Similarly, if you're overweight and turn to food for comfort, you may be feeding an emotional hunger that food cannot satisfy. The truth is, no matter what your body type, balance begins with addressing what has been eating at you, not just what you eat.

Ask yourself: Could your body have been protecting you all along? Is it time to peel away the protective layers and see yourself for who you truly are, beyond your physical form?

Through small yet powerful changes, this 9-week *Stand Up to Slim Down* program will help you shed emotional and physical weight, breaking through old patterns to create a healthier body and mind. You'll release the blocks and barriers holding you back, develop strategies to stay on track, and learn to naturally self-correct behaviors that no longer align with your goals.

Gratitude as Your Foundation

Every journey begins with gratitude. By appreciating where you are and giving thanks at the moment, you create a vortex of energy that empowers your growth. Reflect, meditate, and embrace yourself with love, knowing this positive energy will radiate outward to others.

"It's not what you eat, but what's eating at you that you need to tap into." – Liza

Once you uncover the feelings driving your habits, releasing excess weight becomes easier. Do you agree?

At times, we may feel powerless, as though fate controls our destiny. But the truth is, you have the power to break free from old stories and rewrite your narrative. Even if you've tried before and felt defeated, today is a new day. Stand UP, Step UP, and say YES to yourself. Decide now to **Accept, Appreciate, and Gift Yourself YOU.** I promise to stand by you.

Cause and Effect

Your body is not the cause but the effect, guided by the decisions and beliefs held in your mind. The slightest shift in perception can lead to incredible changes in how you act and react. What once brought you discomfort, grief, or frustration can instead reveal your inner strength and focus.

By aligning your mind with your body's natural intelligence, you can achieve your ideal weight and wellness. When you connect with your core truth, the obstacles standing in your way begin to dissolve.

Your Choice, Your Journey

There are no strict rules in the *Stand Up to Slim Down* program—only choices, and they are yours to make. This booklet is a bridge between your conscious mind and subconscious feelings, offering insights and guidance to help you on this journey. Use the suggestions that resonate with you, and trust that the rest will naturally fall into place.

For deeper support, consider incorporating hypnosis sessions to release underlying emotions. My recordings, such as *Drop Weight* and *Mind-Body Connection,* can help you balance cravings, increase motivation, and accelerate your results. Pair them with *Build Self-Confidence* or *Relax & Unwind* to enhance your transformation.

Live an extraordinary life,
Liza

*"Humans are creatures of habit – we resist change. Yet change is imperative for growth. It's important to push the boundaries of your comfort zone to learn and grow.
That's where the magic happens – You!" ~ Liza*

MY STORY

Greetings, I'm Liza, the founder of HealWithin.com.

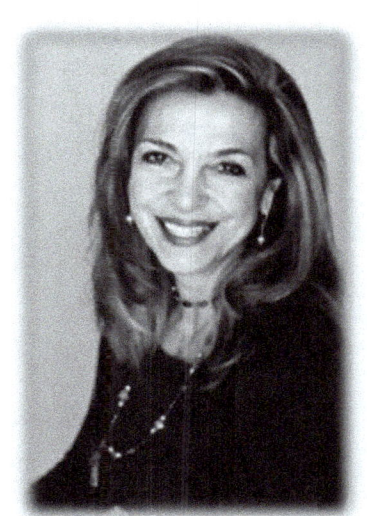

If you're reading this, there's a part of you—whether it's a whisper or a desperate scream—that is searching for change. Maybe it's because you're tired of the weight you carry, physically or emotionally. Maybe it's because you feel stuck, like no matter what you do, the same cycles keep repeating. I see you, and I understand.

Because I've been there.

In 1985, I underwent surgery for an 8.7-centimeter ovarian cyst. A year and a half later, I was back in the operating room for yet another cyst. By 1990, just two years after my second surgery, I found myself sitting in a doctor's office, hearing the same devastating news: another cyst had formed.

By this point, I was divorced, juggling two jobs, and carrying the weight of unrelenting stress and unspoken emotions. I felt exhausted, powerless, and utterly alone.

That day in the doctor's office is seared into my memory. I sat there as he explained that the rapid growth of my previous cysts meant surgery couldn't wait. He recommended we schedule it immediately. As his words sank in, tears welled in my eyes. My throat tightened, and I couldn't speak.

I sat frozen, overwhelmed by fear and hopelessness. My mind flashed back to my last surgery. I remembered lying in the hospital bed, placing my hand on my abdomen, and silently promising myself that the next time I'd enter an operating room, it would be to deliver a baby, not to endure another surgery.

And yet, here I was.

I wanted to cry, to scream, to disappear. But then, something shifted. Somewhere deep inside me, a spark lit—a realization that this moment was a crossroads. I could continue down this path, letting my body bear the brunt of my unspoken pain, or I could take a stand for myself.

I stood up, literally and figuratively. I wiped my tears, placed my feet firmly on the ground, and made a choice: no more.

A Turning Point

With the encouragement of an acupuncturist, I sought out a hypnotherapist. I didn't know what to expect, but I knew I couldn't keep living this way. After just four sessions, my cyst was gone. Gone.

Through those sessions, I discovered something I had never fully understood: my body wasn't working against me—it was protecting me. My cysts were my body's way of screaming for attention, for healing, for release.

For the first time, I began to connect the dots. The stress, the unspoken trauma, the emotions I had buried—they weren't just in my mind; they were stored in my body. My body had been holding the weight of it all, waiting for me to finally listen.

That realization changed everything. It was the moment I understood that what happens *to* us often happens *for* us. My body wasn't my enemy; it was my greatest ally.

Why I'm Sharing This with You

If you're reading this and feeling a pang of recognition, let me tell you this: you're not alone.

You might feel like your body has betrayed you, like you've been carrying a weight that no one else can see. Maybe you've tried everything—diets, exercise, willpower—and still feel stuck. Maybe you've been searching for answers but keep finding dead ends.

I understand that pain, that frustration, that longing for change. And I want you to know it doesn't have to be this way.

"The journey to self-discovery begins when you identify what matters most to you." ~ Liza

A Path to Healing

What I learned through my journey is that true healing begins within. It starts when you pause and listen—not just to your thoughts, but to the wisdom of your body. Your body, mind, heart, and gut are all connected, constantly communicating, and when you learn to align them, miracles happen.

This isn't just about dropping physical weight; it's about releasing the emotional weight you've been carrying for too long. It's about letting go of the patterns and beliefs that no longer serve you. It's about standing up for yourself and choosing to heal, not because you need to be fixed, but because you deserve to feel whole.

My Mission

I left my career in the legal field to become a hypnotherapist because I knew my story wasn't unique. I knew there were countless women like you, carrying invisible burdens, waiting for someone to tell them that healing is possible.

Through HealWithin and the *Stand Up to Slim Down* program, I've dedicated my life to helping women reconnect with their inner power, heal their emotional wounds, and transform their lives.

This program is about more than weight loss—it's about reclaiming yourself. It's about learning to listen to your body, honor your emotions, and step into the life you deserve.

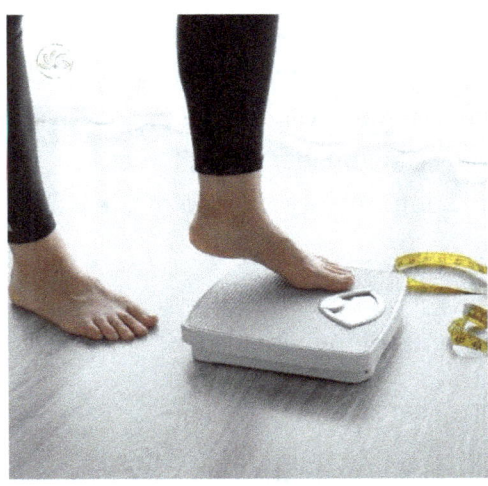

Your Journey Starts Here!

If you've made it here, you've already taken the most crucial step— acknowledging that something needs to change. Now, I invite you to stand up—not just for your body, but for your mind, heart, and spirit. Together, we'll uncover what's been weighing you down, release what no longer serves you, and create a path forward that feels light, joyful, and free.

This program isn't about perfection; it's about progress. It's about embracing yourself with kindness and stepping into the life you deserve. You'll find no starving, no endless cravings, and no struggles here. Instead, you'll discover a process that is **easy, effortless, and even fun** as you watch your body and mind transform over these nine weeks.

Through this journey, you will:

- **Evoke** the patterns and emotions that have kept you stuck.

- **Embrace** your unique self, letting go of the negativity that no longer serves you.

- **Evolve** into a healthier, more aligned version of yourself.

13

This transformation is about more than just releasing physical weight—it's about freeing yourself emotionally, mentally, and spiritually. The lessons in this program will require your active participation. As you practice what you learn, you'll feel empowered, motivated, and supported every step of the way.

Here's What I Know…

Since 1998, I've guided thousands of individuals to:

- Overcome anxiety and fears.

- Shed physical and emotional weight.

- Heal emotional wounds and reclaim their confidence.

But before I could help others, I had to embark on my own healing journey. There was a time when I felt completely out of sync—disconnected from myself, my body, and my purpose. Smoking became my crutch, emotionally eating my escape. I felt trapped in an unhealthy relationship, and my self-esteem was at an all-time low.

Through hypnotherapy, I began to understand that my behaviors weren't failures—they were symptoms. My body wasn't betraying me; it was holding onto emotions and patterns I had ignored for too long. Healing began when I chose to take control, unravel those patterns, and reconnect with myself.

The Truth About Weight

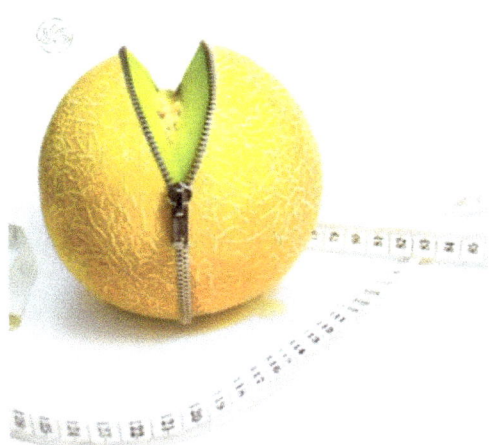

Yes, there are many ways to lose weight. These methods may offer quick fixes, from Ozempic to mushroom coffee to lap band surgery. But let's pause for a moment and consider the message they send to your body: *I hate the way I look. I hate you. I can't stand this.*

This internal negative talk—this cycle of blaming your body—is what truly weighs you down. When you approach weight loss from a place of shame or self-loathing, you're not just fighting your body; you're fighting yourself.

Your body is not the enemy. It is not at fault.

What I offer is different. The *Stand Up to Slim Down* program provides a loving, safe way to connect with your body and yourself truly. It's not about punishing your body or forcing it into submission. It's about listening to its signals, honoring its wisdom, and creating a partnership that nurtures you from the inside out.

If you're fixated on becoming a size 2 at all costs, I'll be honest: you might get there, but at what price? Obsessing over your weight often leads to hating your body, restricting your life, and missing out on joy. That's not what I teach.

Instead, this program will guide you to release weight while cultivating a loving relationship with yourself. When you trust your body and align with its natural wisdom, you unlock the keys to infinite joy, love, possibility, and freedom.

A Safe, Loving Space for Transformation

The *Stand Up to Slim Down* program is a safe and supportive way to release what no longer serves you and step into a healthier, lighter version of yourself. It's designed to meet you exactly where you are and guide you to where you want to go.

Over the years, I've gained and lost weight, but I've learned to accept and love myself through every phase. When I listen to my body's signals—whether it's discomfort after stress eating or the satisfaction of making a nourishing choice—I'm reminded that my body is my greatest ally.

My mission is to help you do the same. To teach you how to stand strong, embrace your unique journey, and confidently say yes to slimming down, not just physically, but emotionally and spiritually.

Progress, Not Perfection

Over the years, I've gained and lost weight. I've quit smoking, only to pick it up again, and then let it go and stop for good. Through it all, I've learned one vital truth: self-compassion is everything.

Today, I don't scold myself for indulging in a treat like ice cream or chocolate. Instead, I trust my body to guide me. I've developed such a deep connection with my body that I can sense its needs, even in the face of stress or emotional challenges. When I overeat or allow stress to linger, my body reacts. It signals me with discomfort, rejecting what doesn't serve me and nudging me to pay attention.

This level of attunement didn't happen overnight—it came from years of learning to listen, honor, and trust my body. Now, I can say "no" without guilt or "yes" without shame, because I know I'm making choices that align with my well-being.

When you learn to *stand up* for yourself, something extraordinary happens. You stop fighting against your body and start working with it. You step into a place of empowerment where you can truly create the life you want.

It Starts with YOU!

This is your moment to stand up, claim your power, and create the life you've been longing for. With every step you take, you'll gain confidence, release old patterns, and reconnect with your body and spirit. You'll discover that your body is not your enemy—it's your ally, guiding you toward health, vitality, and freedom.

The lessons are not just something you will read; doing this program will require your active participation.

There will be **No starving, no cravings, and no more struggles.**

It'll be Easy – Effortless – Even Fun. Just watch your weight drop and transform in 9 weeks!

Join my clients who already know the secret to Healing Within! Become part of the bigger healing circle – empowering yourself and motivating others! Ask to join our private FB group.

To celebrate the new you, you must be fearless and bold, learn to tap within, and declare your intentions. It is time you retrain yourself to stop negative talks, validate emotions of fears in their tracks, and Stand Up to... evoke your passion, embrace your femininity, and evolve spiritually.

- Take ownership of what you evoke – it is realized.
- Take ownership of what you embrace - you validate.
- Take ownership of what you evolve to - a healthier and loving person, a better lifestyle.
  Because... You Matter

What You'll Discover

In this program, you'll uncover the mental, emotional, and physical weight you've been carrying—and learn how to release it. You'll understand how to care for yourself in a way that honors your mind, body, and spirit. When you do, your body will naturally shift into its ideal shape and size for your unique constitution, lifestyle, and age. For some, this might mean dropping a few sizes. For others, it's about learning to love the body you're in right now. Regardless of your goal, by committing to this program, you'll gain confidence and feel more beautiful, sexy, and comfortable with yourself than you have in years.

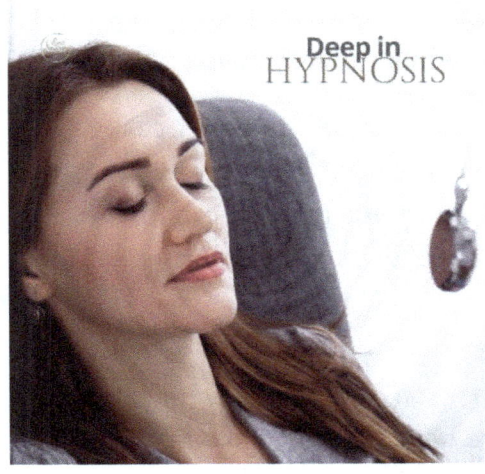

WHAT IS HYPNOSIS?

Understanding Hypnosis

Wikipedia defines hypnosis as "a human condition involving focused attention."

When you hear the word *hypnosis,* what comes to mind? Do you picture a stage hypnotist entertaining an audience, making volunteers bark like dogs, dancing awkwardly, or performing silly acts? Or do you think of it as a tool for quitting smoking or losing weight?

For most people, hypnosis feels like a mystery. There's a curiosity about what it truly is, but also a hesitation, rooted in misconceptions from Hollywood movies or dramatic stage shows.

Here's the truth: hypnosis isn't about losing control. In fact, it's the opposite—it's about gaining clarity and focus by accessing the deeper parts of your mind. Hypnosis is a natural state, something you've already experienced countless times without realizing it.

Have you ever become so lost in a book or movie that the world around you disappeared? Or driven somewhere only to realize you don't remember much of the drive? Perhaps you've calmed a crying child with a kiss and the assurance, "It's all better now." These are all examples of natural hypnotic states.

Hypnosis isn't strange, magical, or mysterious—it's calming, relaxing, and deeply pleasant. You don't go *under* hypnosis; you go *into* hypnosis. This state allows you to focus inward, unlocking the immense potential of your mind and body.

> *"If you think you can – you can. And if you think you can't, you are right!"* ~ Mary Kay Ash

The Power of Hypnosis

Hypnosis is a tool—an incredibly powerful one—that allows you to harness the potential of your subconscious mind. In the hypnotic state, you can focus your attention on specific goals or challenges, accessing the part of your mind that controls your habits, emotions, and beliefs.

Think of your subconscious as a garden. Every thought, belief, and experience is a seed planted in the soil. Some seeds grow into beautiful, life-affirming habits, while others—planted in moments of pain, fear, or doubt—become weeds that choke out your potential.

The Conscious and Subconscious Minds

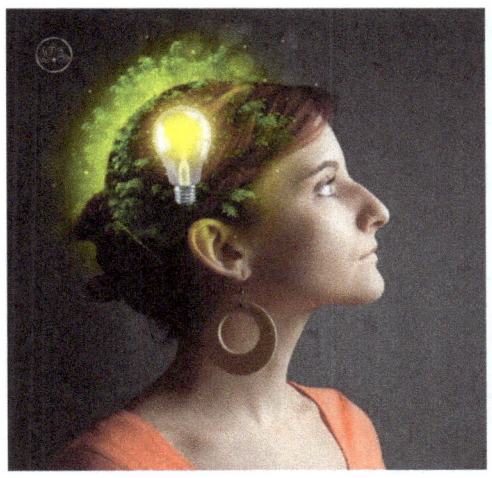

To truly understand hypnosis, you need to understand the two parts of your mind: the conscious and the subconscious.

The conscious mind is the logical, analytical part of you. It's the voice in your head that says, "I should stop smoking," or "I need to lose weight." It's also where willpower resides, which is why you might feel strong and motivated one moment, only to give in to temptation the next.

The subconscious mind, on the other hand, is where real power lies. It's the storehouse of your emotions, habits, memories, and instincts. It governs involuntary functions like breathing and heart rate, and it accepts everything it's told as truth. The subconscious mind doesn't argue or analyze—it simply acts on the programming it's received over time.

When these two parts of your mind are out of sync—when your conscious mind says, "I want to change," but your subconscious holds onto old habits—it creates internal conflict. Hypnosis serves as a bridge, bypassing the critical filter between the two, so you can reprogram your subconscious and create lasting change.

Feeding Your Subconscious

Your subconscious mind doesn't judge. It simply accepts what it's told. This is why early childhood experiences have such a profound impact on our habits and behaviors as adults.

Think about this: a child falls off their bike and cries. A parent rushes to comfort them with a cookie, saying, "Here, this will make you feel better." The child learns to associate food with comfort. As they grow, they might not consciously remember that moment, but the pattern remains: when they feel emotional pain, they turn to food for relief.

The *Stand Up to Slim Down* program helps you break these patterns by addressing their root causes. By reprogramming your subconscious, you can create a healthier, more empowering relationship with food and your body.

Hypnosis helps you tend to this garden. It allows you to pull out the weeds and nurture the seeds that align with your goals. Through this process, you can:

- Break free from habits like smoking or overeating.
- Overcome fears and anxieties.
- Build self-esteem and confidence.
- Improve sleep, focus, and athletic performance.
- Create a healthier relationship with food and your body.

What Does Hypnosis Feel Like?

When people learn I'm a clinical hypnotherapist, they often ask, "What does it feel like?"

Hypnosis feels different for everyone. For some, it's a deep, meditative state where they feel weightless and free. For others, it's a light relaxation, like daydreaming. It's not about how "deep" you go—it's about your ability to focus inward and connect with your subconscious mind.

One of my clients described their first experience with hypnosis:

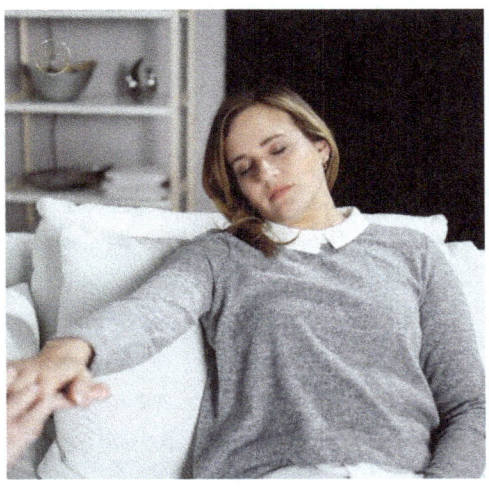

A Client's Experience

"I remember quite clearly the first time I was hypnotized. I was referred to Liza for panic and anxiety, and I was also told I needed to lose over 20 pounds. I had been curious about hypnosis for many years, wondering how it worked and if it could truly help me. Honestly, my curiosity about how Liza could help me lose weight and overcome my panic was a huge factor in deciding to see her.

"Sitting in her recliner, she asked me to focus on a spot and close my eyes whenever I was ready. Inwardly, I was nervous, thinking, 'I don't really know her, and here I am surrendering all my control in a place I've never been to before.' But I quickly reasoned with myself—I had chosen to trust her.

"I closed my eyes, and almost immediately, I could feel my heart beating faster. Paranoid thoughts crept into my mind. I had never seen a demonstration of hypnotherapy before. The only hypnosis I had ever witnessed was stage hypnosis, where people did silly things like cluck like chickens. I wondered, 'What if she makes me do or say something embarrassing?' My curiosity turned into apprehension.

"I opened my eyes slightly and slyly peeped around. Liza smiled warmly at me as if she knew what I was thinking. That smile reassured me. I let my eyes close again and began listening to her words.

"Her voice was slow and comforting, occasionally dropping to a whisper. She started by asking me to focus on my breathing, guiding me to take slow, deep breaths. Almost immediately, I felt my heart begin to slow, and I started to relax.

"She spoke of becoming aware of my body, imagining myself walking down steps, and feeling more deeply relaxed with each step. Each time she said the words 'deeper relax,' I felt a wave of calm wash over me, flowing from my head to my toes. I thought, 'This is all right. I feel safe.'

"But then, my logical mind kicked in: 'I can still hear her. I know exactly where I am. Is this it? Is this what hypnosis feels like?' I felt comfortable and relaxed, but I was a little disappointed that nothing 'magical' seemed to be happening. Then, after reflecting for a few moments, I realized something important— I didn't *want* anything magical to happen. What I truly wanted was to feel safe, calm, and in control.

"Still, my mind couldn't help but challenge itself: 'Maybe something magical *is* happening. How do I know I can still move my hand? What if the control I think I have is just an illusion?' I decided to test it. I twitched the fingers on my left hand, just slightly. They moved! I felt a sense of relief and comfort knowing that no one was in control of me but me.

"That realization shattered my warped perception of hypnosis but also brought me so much peace. I thought to myself, 'This feels like meditation.' I knew I could stand up and walk out of the room at any time—just as Liza had assured me.

"Then something unexpected happened. Liza began counting me back up: 'Five, four, three, two, one, and fully wide awake.' My mind felt as though it was gently lifted back into full awareness. I blinked my eyes open, scanning the room with a slightly glazed expression. My hands felt a little numb and cool, but I felt... amazing.

"When I glanced at the clock, I was stunned. Fifty minutes had passed, but it felt like only five. I had never felt so calm and relaxed in my entire life. Nothing weird or 'magical' had happened, but somehow, it worked. I felt calm, grounded, and at ease.

"As I drove the 14 miles back home, I had plenty of time to process the session. I realized that I had walked into Liza's office with so many misconceptions about hypnosis, misconceptions shaped by stage shows, and old black-and-white movies where hypnotists-controlled people's minds with a pocket watch or a piercing stare. By the end of the day, I realized that hypnotherapy wasn't about power or control. It was about collaboration—relaxing the mind and allowing Liza to guide me toward the changes I wanted to make. Hypnosis wasn't something being done *to* me—it was something I was doing *with* her help.

"I also learned something else that day: most people naturally enter hypnotic states several times a day without realizing it. Although everyone's experience of hypnosis is personal and unique, I hope I've been able to share some insight into what it feels like.

"For anyone considering hypnosis as a therapeutic option, I hope this puts your mind at ease. A hypnotic trance is simply a natural, relaxed state of mind that almost anyone can achieve. You are still you, and you are still in control.

"And if you're working with someone like Liza, you're in very capable, loving hands. Enjoy the journey!"

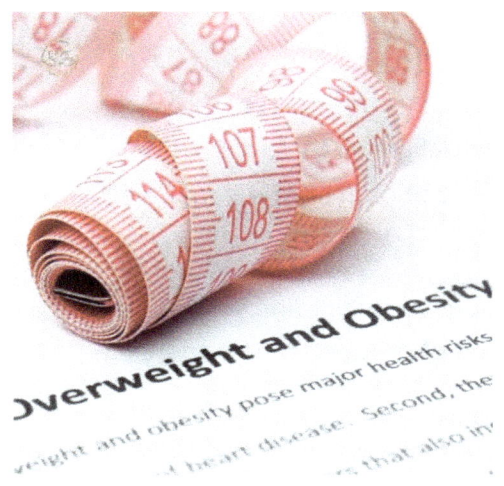

Overweight and Obesity

...verweight and obesity pose major health risks ...eight and obesity pose major health risks. Second, the ... heart disease. ... that also in...

Breaking the Cycle

Do you catch yourself saying, "I hate the way I look," or "I can't stand my body"? These aren't just fleeting thoughts, they're planted in your subconscious. Words have power. When repeated, they shape how you see yourself and how your body responds to you.

This program will teach you how to reframe these thoughts into affirmations that heal and uplift. Instead of saying, "I hate my fat stomach," try, "I've been storing energy here—it's time to release what I no longer need and care for myself."

Changing your inner dialogue aligns your conscious and subconscious minds. This shift not only nurtures self-love but also paves the way for lasting transformation.

Your Journey to Wholeness

This program isn't just about shedding pounds. It's about shedding the emotional weight of old stories, limiting beliefs, and self-doubt. Together, we'll explore the deeper reasons behind your eating habits, reprogram your subconscious, and cultivate a loving relationship with your body.

Here's what you'll gain:

- Confidence in your body and yourself.
- Healthier habits that align with your goals.
- Freedom from the emotional burdens that weigh you down.

This is your journey to wholeness. By feeding your soul with kindness, you'll discover a life of empowerment and ease.

This program will guide you to:

- Recognize and release negative beliefs about food and your body.
- Build confidence and self-esteem.
- Embrace healthier habits and let go of what no longer serves you.

Feed your soul with kindness, and watch the struggles fade away.

Are you now ready to stand up for yourself?

You deserve to feel whole, empowered, and free.

USES FOR HYPNOSIS: You can use hypnosis to:

- ✓ improve memory, concentration, and study habits
- ✓ rid yourself of habits such as smoking, overeating or nail-biting
- ✓ control urges and weight
- ✓ boost self-esteem and confidence
- ✓ improve sleep patterns and athletic abilities
- ✓ reduce stress and anxiety
- ✓ overcome fears and phobias, speaking in public, etc.
- ✓ reduce pain
- ✓ Create better habits – create healthier choices and patterns in mind and body.

In hypnosis, you are always in control – even though it appears as if you have no control.

Through the "Stand Up to Slim Down Program," I help you...

- Build up your confidence and self-esteem so you can accept a thinner self;
- Experience dropping the unwanted weight;
- Maintain your desired weight;
- Incorporate new habits into your life
- Recognize past patterns and give less importance to negative chatter;
- Increase the appeal of healthier foods to be more desirable and fatty foods less desirable;
- Incorporate healthier patterns of behavior regarding food, people, and reasons.

Important note: Behind many unhealthy eating habits is a hidden fear. And until that fear is faced and released, the weight it causes won't fully let go—no matter how hard you try.

The subconscious mind cannot distinguish between a wish and a fear. If and when fear dominates your thinking, that thinking becomes a wish that the subconscious mind attempts to bring into reality. The subconscious never sleeps, never ceases to operate, and keeps you going with your voluntary and involuntary actions. Once the subconscious mind accepts an idea, it begins to make the idea a reality. It works the same for good or bad ideas. When applied negatively, the subconscious can be the cause of failure, frustration, unhappiness, and even illness.

Your subconscious mind is like the soil that accepts any seeds, good or bad. It is the seed of your emotions and the storehouse of your memory.

You move towards your most dominant thought pattern. So, if you are worried about or fear something, STOP whenever that fear or worry comes to your mind. Think about how you can say the same thing more lovingly and positively. Soon, you'll become accustomed to thinking positively.

Instead of saying, "I hate the way I look," change it to…
"How can I be kinder to my body and myself? What can I do to feel good about myself?" "I can't stand my fat stomach and body" to "I've been storing some fat here - time to do something about it."

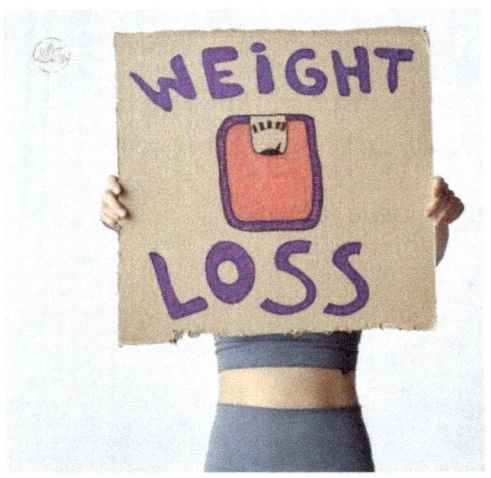

The Subconscious Mind, Weight, and Your Body

Your subconscious mind is a powerful ally. It holds the beliefs that shape your actions, often working behind the scenes. If food has been your comfort or escape, your subconscious sees it as a solution, whether or not it's helpful.

This program will help you reprogram those patterns by:

- Releasing emotional attachments to food.
- Building healthier, sustainable habits.
- Replacing self-criticism with self-compassion.

When your mind and body align, transformation becomes natural and lasting. Right now, you might feel disconnected from your body. Maybe you've felt betrayed by its appearance, its weight, or its limitations. But here's the truth: your body is not your enemy. It aims to protect you, guide you, and support you—even when it feels like it's doing the opposite.

The Power of Self-Talk

Take a moment to think about the last thing you said to yourself about your body. Was it kind? Or was it critical?

For many women, this inner dialogue is harsh:

- "I can't stand the way I look."

- "I'll never lose this weight."

- "Why can't I look like her?"

Your subconscious mind hears these words as commands. It doesn't distinguish between fleeting thoughts and deeply held beliefs. It simply listens, accepts, and acts.

When you criticize your body, it responds. Your muscles tense, your energy drops, and your posture collapses under the weight of those words. But when you speak kindly to yourself, your body aligns with that energy. It listens, heals, and moves toward balance.

The Subconscious Mind and Your Core

Your subconscious mind is the control center of your body. It regulates your breathing, digestion, and heartbeat without conscious thought. It also holds your beliefs about yourself—beliefs that shape how you see your body and how your body responds.

If you've spent years thinking, "I'm not good enough," or "I'll always struggle with my weight," your subconscious mind works to align your behaviors with those beliefs. It isn't punishing you—it's following the programming it's been given.

Now imagine shifting that programming. When you begin to believe, "I can nourish and care for my body," or "I deserve to feel healthy and strong," your subconscious aligns your actions with those beliefs. You start making choices that reflect love and respect for yourself.

Rebuilding a Loving Relationship with Your Body

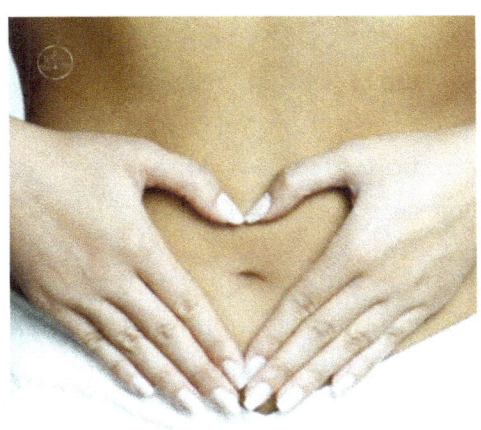

Your body aims to support you in every way it can. It wants to heal, to balance itself, and to thrive. But it needs your partnership. The relationship you have with your body is just like any other relationship—it requires care, respect, and communication.

Here's how to rebuild that connection:

1. **Listen to Your Body**
   Your body communicates with you constantly. Hunger, fatigue, discomfort, and even cravings are all messages. Instead of ignoring or silencing these signals, pause and ask, "What do I need right now?" Honor your body's wisdom.

2. **Transform Your Inner Dialogue**
   Each time you catch yourself in negative self-talk, stop.
   Replace it with loving, constructive words. For example:

   - Instead of "I hate my stomach," say, "My body is
     learning to let go of what no longer serves me."

   - Instead of "I'll never lose weight," say, "I am
     creating a healthier relationship with my body
     every day."

3. **Release Stored Emotions**
   Through practices like deep breathing, movement, and
   hypnosis, you can release the emotional weight stored
   in your body. These emotions aren't weaknesses—they
   are signals, asking to be seen and released.

4. **Reconnect with Your Core**
   Your core is more than your physical center. It's where
   your emotions, intuition, and strength reside. Spend
   time each day reconnecting with this part of yourself
   through mindfulness, visualization, or movement.

Did You Know Your Muscles Have Memory?

Muscle memory isn't just about recalling how to ride a bike or
nail that dance move you practiced endlessly in the '90s (yes,
your Electric Slide still counts!). Your muscles are like tiny
librarians, keeping records of every fall, every stretch, and even
every time you overdid it at the gym because "leg day" felt like
a good idea.

But here's where it gets fascinating—and a little unfair. Muscles also remember emotional experiences. Ever notice how your shoulders creep up to your ears during a stressful meeting? Or how your jaw suddenly feels tighter than your skinny jeans after the holidays? That's your muscles holding onto tension, stress, and unprocessed emotions like overzealous hoarders.

The good news? Just as muscles can learn to react protectively, they can also relearn to let go. Through mindful movement, deep breathing, and a good laugh (seriously, laughter is a great release!), you can retrain your body to loosen up and embrace freedom.

So next time you catch yourself clenching, remind your muscles: "Hey, we're not auditioning for a tension convention!" Your body is always speaking to you—sometimes with a whisper, sometimes with a scream. Are you ready to tune in?

Muscle Memory and Emotional Imprints

Your muscles aren't just physical—they're emotional record-keepers. They store tension, stress, and memories, much like little librarians cataloging every experience.

Ever notice how your shoulders tighten during stress, or your chest feels heavy with sadness? These aren't random. They're your body holding onto emotional energy.

The good news? Your muscles can learn to let go. Through mindful movement, deep breathing, and even a good laugh, you can release these imprints and embrace freedom.

So next time you catch yourself clenching your jaw or hunching your shoulders, pause. Take a deep breath and remind your body, "It's okay to let go now."

But your body also has an incredible capacity to release and heal. By addressing the emotional imprints stored within, you can let go of the weight—both physical and emotional—that has been holding you back.

Your body isn't your enemy; it's your greatest ally. To rebuild this partnership, you need to treat it with care, respect, and kindness.

Here's how to start:

1. **Listen to Your Body**
   Your body communicates through hunger, discomfort, and cravings. Pause and ask, "What do I really need right now?" Honor its wisdom.

2. **Transform Your Inner Dialogue**
    Catch negative self-talk and replace it with loving affirmations:

    o   Instead of "I hate my thighs," say, "I'm grateful for my strong legs that carry me through life."

3. **Release Stored Emotions**
    Use practices like deep breathing, movement, and hypnosis to let go of emotional tension stored in your muscles.

4. **Reconnect with Your Core**
    Your core is more than physical strength—it's where your emotions and intuition reside. Spend time reconnecting with this part of yourself through mindfulness or movement.

Speaking Kindly to Your Body

Imagine talking to your body as if it were a dear friend. Would you say, "I hate you," or "You're not good enough"? Of course not. You would say, "Thank you for carrying me," or "I appreciate you for all that you do."

Although this may seem awkward, this exercise can shift your relationship with your body:

- **Write a Love Letter**: Thank your body for its strength, resilience, and support. Apologize for the times you've been critical. Commit to speaking kindly and caring for it.

- **Practice Gratitude**: Each day, list three things you're grateful for about your body. For example:
    - "I'm grateful for my legs—they carry me through my day."
    - "I'm grateful for my lungs—they allow me to breathe deeply and fully."
    - "I'm grateful for my heart—it beats faithfully for me every moment."

- **Affirm Your Worth**: Use affirmations to guide your subconscious toward healing. Repeat phrases like:
    - "I am creating a loving relationship with my body."
    - "My body is my partner in health and happiness."
    - "I release what no longer serves me."

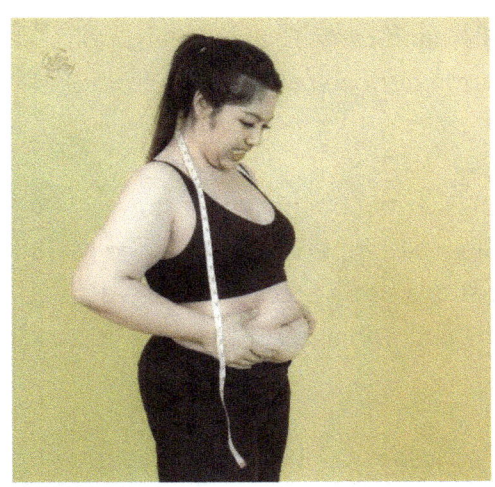

Your Body Listens

Every thought you think, every word you speak, and every feeling you hold is heard by your body. It responds not out of punishment, but out of alignment with your thoughts and beliefs.

When you choose to speak lovingly to your body, to honor its needs, and to treat it with care, you create a powerful shift. Your body aligns with your intentions, and together, you begin to release the weight of old patterns, stories, and emotions.

This isn't just about shedding pounds. It's about creating harmony between your mind, body, and spirit. It's about learning to celebrate yourself, not for what you hope to become, but for who you already are.

Here are some statistics.

According to the CDC, the prevalence of obesity in the United States between 2015-2016 was 39.6%. This means that almost 40% of adults in the US are obese.

According to the Centers for Disease Control and Prevention (CDC), between August 2021 and August 2023, the prevalence of obesity among adults in the U.S. was 40.3%. This is a slight decrease from the 41.9% reported between 2017 and 2020, but the change is not statistically significant. The prevalence of severe obesity during the same period was 9.4%, up from 7.7% in 2013–2014. ?

Regarding children and adolescents, the most recent data available from the CDC indicates that between 2017 and March 2020, the prevalence of obesity among adolescents aged 12–19 years was 22.2%, and among children aged 6–11 years, it was 20.7%.

According to the Centers for Disease Control and Prevention (CDC), between August 2021 and August 2023, the prevalence of obesity among adults in the U.S. was 40.3%. This is a slight decrease from the 41.9% reported between 2017 and 2020, but the change is not statistically significant.

The prevalence of severe obesity during the same period was 9.4%, up from 7.7% in 2013–2014. Regarding children and adolescents, the most recent data available from the CDC indicates that between 2017 and March 2020, the prevalence of obesity among adolescents aged 12–19 years was 22.2%, and among children aged 6–11 years, it was 20.7%.

Breaking the Cycle: For You and Your Children

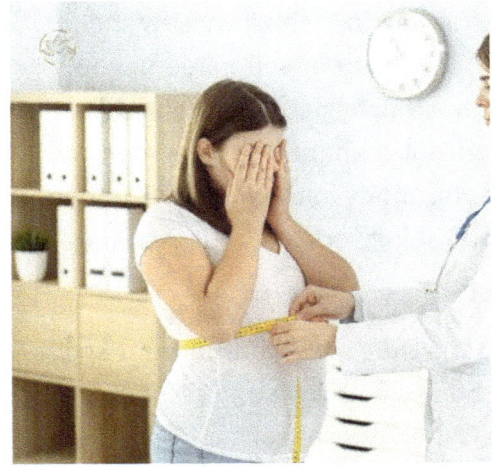

If you've struggled with weight or body image, you're not alone. For many women, these struggles began in childhood. Maybe you were teased by other kids or endured unkind comments from family members. Perhaps you were told you weren't good enough, pretty enough, or thin enough to fit in. Those words don't just sting at the moment—they stay with you, embedding themselves in your subconscious and shaping the way you see yourself for years to come.

Now, as an adult, you may still carry those wounds. And if you're a parent, there's a chance those same patterns are showing up in your children.

These figures highlight the ongoing challenge of obesity. This isn't just about numbers. It's about real people—adults and children, just like many of us—carrying not only physical weight but the emotional weight of societal pressure, self-criticism, and sometimes even bullying.

The Legacy of Body Image

As parents, we set the tone for how our children view their bodies. If you've struggled with weight or self-esteem, you might worry about passing those struggles on to your kids. It's not just what you say to them—it's what they observe in you. Do they hear you criticizing your body in the mirror? Do they see you skipping meals or punishing yourself with extreme diets?

Children learn by watching, and they absorb far more than we realize. When we treat our bodies with love and respect, we teach them to do the same. When we break free from the cycle of self-criticism and emotional eating, we empower ourselves to grow up with a healthier relationship with food and our bodies.

Why This Program Matters

The *Stand Up to Slim Down* program isn't just about you—it's about breaking the cycle for future generations. It's about understanding the connection between mind and body and teaching your children to do the same. When you heal your relationship with your body, you permit your kids to approach theirs with curiosity and kindness instead of shame.

This program gives you tools not only to improve your health but also to help your children:

- Understand their bodies: Teach them to listen to their physical and emotional needs.

- Break free from harmful patterns: Help them recognize the difference between emotional and physical hunger.

- Build self-esteem: Show them how to speak kindly to themselves and celebrate their unique qualities.

- Create healthier habits: Model behaviors that prioritize nourishment, movement, and self-care over restriction and punishment.

Your journey isn't just about dropping pounds or changing your appearance. It's about creating a ripple effect that transforms not only your life but the lives of those around you.

When you take steps to heal within, you pave the way for your children to grow up with confidence, self-awareness, and a deep connection to their own bodies. You're not just standing up for yourself—you're standing up for them, too.

And here's something else to consider:

Our children are growing up in a world that bombards them with conflicting messages about beauty, body size, self-worth, and what it means to be "enough." Social media, peer pressure, and even school environments can create insecurities long before a child fully understands who they are. That's why what happens at home becomes the foundation of their emotional resilience.

When your child sees you pause before reacting to your reflection...
When they witness you enjoying a meal with gratitude instead of guilt...

When they hear you speak kindly to yourself after a hard day...
They are not just witnessing habits—they are absorbing values.

This is how healing becomes a legacy.
By showing up for yourself, you show them what self-respect
looks like in action.
By choosing grace over shame, you teach them that their worth
isn't defined by appearance.

The work you're doing here matters more than you may realize.
It's not just about creating a healthier relationship with food
and your body; it's about becoming a living example of
compassion, strength, and possibility.

So, if guilt ever sneaks in... if you ever think, "Why didn't I do
this sooner?" Please remember: you're doing it now. And now
is exactly the right time.

Each conscious step you take, each pattern you break—is a gift.
A gift to yourself.
And a powerful inheritance for those who come after you.

This is your time.
To rise.
To reset.
To reframe the future—not only for you, but for your children
and their children.

Let's make this journey one that reshapes not just your body
but your legacy.

Because when you heal... they learn to thrive.

The Power of 9: Completion

As you approach this program, keep in mind that 9 is the number of completion and birthing. By the end of this program, you'll have gone through all three phases:

1. **Evoking:** Bringing the subconscious to the surface.

2. **Embracing:** Accepting, validating, and loving all parts of yourself.

3. **Evolving:** Stepping into the person you've always been meant to be.

Let's lean into this journey with gratitude, excitement, and an open heart.

Are you now ready to embark on a journey toward becoming healthier and lighter in soul, mind, and body?

We start with the soul because it resides within the body. The soul speaks to the mind, the mind communicates with the body, and the heart connects it all.

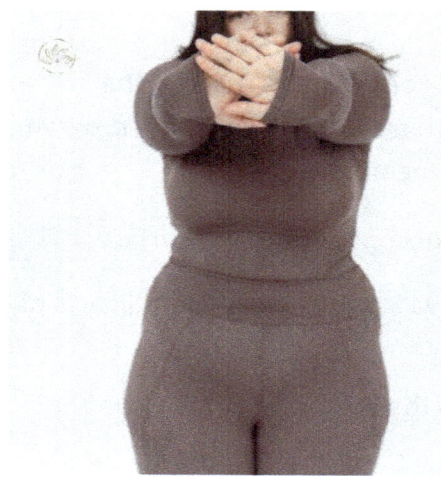

WEEK ONE - Begin Your Change!

Why Stand Up to Slim Down?

Welcome! By starting this program, you've already taken the most important step: showing up for yourself. Congratulations on saying "yes" to your transformation. It's not just about weight loss—it's about reclaiming your power, health, and joy. Think of this as your Stand-Up moment—the one where you decide to stop playing small and start showing up fully—mind, body, and spirit.

Many women, including me, have carried the burden of emotional, physical, and mental weight. That weight isn't just on our bodies—it's in our hearts, our minds, and our stories. For years, I thought I had to fix my body to fix my life. But I discovered something profound: change starts within. When you reconnect with your mind, body, and core, everything— and I mean everything—begins to shift.

This program is not about perfection. It's about freedom. It's about honoring who you are – your story, evoking the emotions buried deep within, embracing every part of you as you are today, and evolving into the lighter, freer version of yourself.

46

Why "Drop" Weight Instead of "Lose" Weight?

Words are powerful. They shape our thoughts, influence our emotions, and direct our actions. When you say, "I want to lose weight," it can trigger resistance in your subconscious mind. Losing something implies deprivation or the potential for regret. Who wants to lose something they value—even if it's weight?

Instead, think of weight as something you're ready to drop. Like shedding an old coat on a warm spring day or letting go of a heavy bag you've carried far too long. Dropping weight is a conscious choice, a release of what no longer serves you, and a step toward freedom.

What else are you ready to drop?

- Self-doubt?

- Old patterns that held you back?

- The belief that you're not worthy of the transformation you desire.

This program isn't just about weight—it's about releasing the emotional and mental burdens you've carried, creating space for a healthier, more vibrant you.

Your Words Shape Your World Starting today, replace "lose weight" with "drop weight." Notice how it feels lighter, more intentional, and empowering.

Story: Meet Carla

Carla came to me frustrated. "I've tried every diet out there, and nothing works," she said during our first session. She felt defeated, stuck in a cycle of guilt and shame. But as we worked together, she uncovered the real reason she struggled: she'd spent years putting everyone else first—her kids, her job, her friends. She'd been giving from an empty cup. Once Carla realized this, her mindset shifted. Week by week, she started setting small boundaries, like saying "no" without guilt and carving out time for herself. The weight? It began to drop, but more importantly, Carla felt lighter in spirit.

What about you? Are you ready to prioritize yourself?

Your Why Matters

Before we go any further, let's pause and reflect deeply:

- Why do you truly want to drop the weight?

- How many pounds would you release to feel lighter, not just in your body, but in your spirit?

- How many times have you ridden the yo-yo cycle of gain, loss, and gain again?

Is your goal to:

- Feel more confident in your own skin?

- Reclaim your health, energy, and vitality.

- Break free from the stories, habits, or cycles that no longer serve you.

Your why is your compass—it's the foundation for every step you'll take in this program. It's what will guide you when the path feels challenging or unclear.

And remember, this is *your* journey. You are not in competition with anyone else. Let go of the comparisons and embrace *your* truth, *your* needs, and *your* dreams. This is about *you*.

Evoking Your Story

Let's begin by evoking what was. Your story matters. The beliefs, patterns, and experiences that have shaped your relationship with your body are important to acknowledge.

Think back to your earliest memories of your body and food. Were you praised for being small? Teased for being big? Did food represent love, comfort, or celebration? Or was it a source of guilt, shame, or control?

For many women, weight becomes a shield—a way to feel safe, a way to protect ourselves from hurt or judgment. Other times, it becomes a punishment, a way to hold on to guilt or shame. These stories are not your reality—they are simply the past. And by evoking them, you gain the power to release them.

Take a moment to reflect on the following:

- What messages did I receive about my body growing up?
- How did my family talk about food, weight, or beauty?
- When I think about my weight, what emotions surface?

Write your thoughts freely. Let them flow without judgment. This is your space to honor what was.

The Connection Between Mind, Body, and Core

Your body is more than just a vessel. It's a sacred home for your mind and spirit. When you speak negatively about your body, every cell, every muscle, and every organ feels it. Your body is always listening.

Have you ever noticed how your body reacts to stress? How does your stomach knot with anxiety or your shoulders tense with fear? Your body carries memories—not just in your mind but in your muscles and tissues. This is why self-talk matters.

Instead of saying, "I hate the way I look," ask yourself, "How can I show my body more love today?"

Your body is not your enemy. It's your partner. It has been with you through every triumph and every challenge. By reconnecting with your core—your mind-brain, heart-brain, and gut-brain—you can begin to release the weight of what no longer serves you.

Let's Lighten Things Up

Weight loss is like a GPS. Sometimes you take a detour (like enjoying a late-night bowl of ice cream), but if you recalibrate, you'll still arrive at your destination. And yes, if your "destination" includes comfort and ease, even in stretchy pants, remember—it's about feeling good, not judgment.

Understanding Emotional Weight

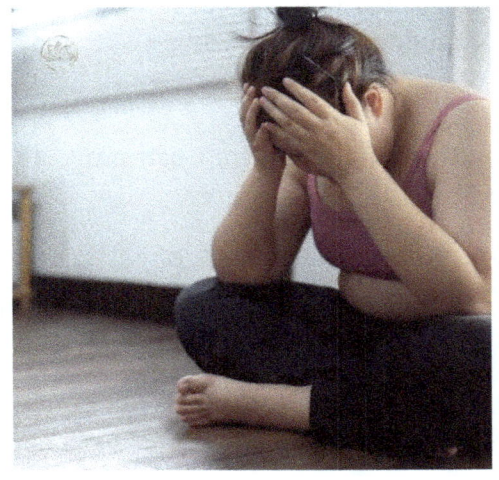

For many of us, weight isn't just about what we eat. It's about what's eating at us. Stress, trauma, heartbreak, and unprocessed emotions can manifest physically.

Your body responds to these internal battles with protection mechanisms—holding onto weight as if to shield you from the world.

Consider these common causes of emotional weight:

- **Safety:** Does extra weight make you feel less vulnerable?

- **Protection:** Is your body keeping you safe by holding onto pain or past trauma?

- **Stress:** Do you use food to cope with the pressures of life?

- **Menopause/Post-Pregnancy:** Are hormonal changes affecting your weight and self-image?

These questions aren't easy, but they're necessary. When you bring these emotions to light, you begin the process of letting them go.

Why Weight Won't Stay Off?

Let's be honest: You've probably lost weight before.
You've followed the plans, skipped the sugar, worked out, and seen some results.
But then... life happened.
The weight returned. The motivation faded. The frustration built up again.

This cycle, what we call **yo-yo weight**, is not a lack of willpower. It's a signal. A deep, subconscious pattern that is still running the show.

You see, part of you wants to move forward. You envision feeling light, confident, beautiful, walking into a room, and being seen and celebrated.
But then there's another part of you—quiet, hidden, and deeply protective—that pulls you right back into the familiar.

That part of you lives in the subconscious. And its job is not to make you skinny, happy, or successful.
Its job is to keep you safe.

Even if that "safety" means staying stuck.

Here's an example I've seen often in my clients—and even in myself:
You might consciously say, *"I want to look good. I want to be slim. I want to feel beautiful."*
But underneath that, there might be a belief formed way back in childhood, like:

- *Pretty girls are mean.*
- *Skinny girls are selfish.*
- *If I'm attractive, I'll be judged.*
- *If I lose weight, I'll be visible—and visibility isn't safe.*

Maybe you were once excluded by a group of "beautiful" girls in school—the blond, rich, confident girls who seemed to have it all. You might have felt rejected, unworthy, or even angry. Your subconscious mind stored that pain and formed a belief to protect you:

Better to stay hidden than risk being hurt again.

You didn't even know this belief was there.
Until one day, through hypnotherapy, you connected the dots. And you realized that the little girl inside of you was just trying to protect you.

But what kept you safe back then may be holding you back now. That's why this program begins **not with restriction or dieting**, but with awareness.
The first step is not shrinking your body; it's understanding your story.

Through guided techniques, self-reflection, and subconscious work, we begin to untangle those deeply rooted beliefs. We replace fear with truth. We honor the younger version of you who needed protection... while giving the woman you are today the power to choose differently.

This week, ask yourself:

- What am I really afraid might happen if I lose weight?
- Who might I become if I step out of hiding?
- What beliefs did I pick up as a child that may no longer be true today?

Because until you change the **inner narrative**, the outer results won't last.

Let this week be the beginning of a new dialogue—with your body, your subconscious, and your true self.

Let's *evoke* what's been running beneath the surface so we can *embrace* your truth and *evolve* with clarity, compassion, and courage.

You are not broken.
You are not weak.
You've just been protecting yourself.

Your Week One Checklist

1. **Commit to the Journey:** Write a short affirmation to guide you this week. Example: "I choose to prioritize myself because I deserve to feel vibrant and strong."

2. **Identify Your Triggers:** What situations or emotions make you reach for food when you're not hungry? Write them down.

3. **Small Wins:** Set one small, achievable goal for the week. Example: Drink a glass of water before each meal or take a 10-minute walk daily.

Your Commitment to YOU!

Take a moment to pause and reflect on your decision to begin. It's okay if it feels overwhelming; big changes always do. You may say I have done this many times before... It's OK. Let's do this together!

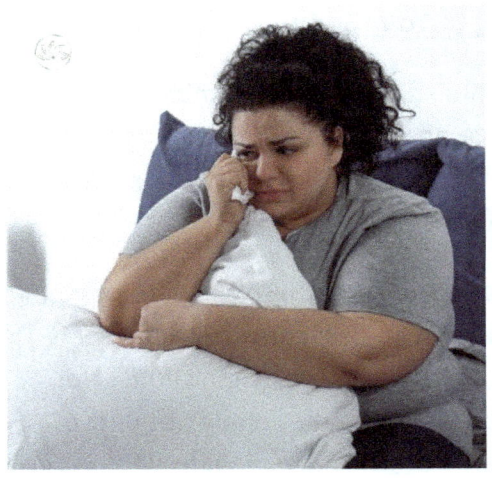

WEEK TWO - Discovering Your Patterns

Week Two: Discovering Your Patterns

Welcome to Week Two! This week, we embark on an exciting journey of self-discovery. By understanding the patterns and habits that have shaped your relationship with food, we unlock the keys to transformation. Let's gently peel back the layers, step by step, to uncover the truth about what drives your choices and how to realign them with your goals.

Why Your Words Matter

Words matter. When you say, "I want to lose weight," your subconscious mind might resist. After all, who wants to lose anything? Dropping weight, on the other hand, implies a choice, like letting go of an old sweater that no longer fits. It's freeing, not depriving.

Think about it: What else can you let go of that no longer serves you? Negative self-talk, old habits, or even that box of stale cookies in the pantry?

A New Approach: Listening to Your Body

In this program, we take a holistic approach, combining facts, science, emotional coaching, healthy eating, affirmations, and imagery. It's not about restriction or punishment—it's about ease, grace, and alignment.

Imagine this: You're at a gathering, and there's a plate of your former go-to comfort food. Instead of feeling powerless or tempted, you calmly pass it by, saying, "No, thank you." Not out of force or willpower, but because it's simply not part of the "new you." It's effortless, natural, and freeing.

You're not unhealthy deep down. Your subconscious mind is your greatest ally. As children, our bodies intuitively know what they need. Have you ever seen a baby spit out food they dislike or stop eating when they're full? That's the body's innate wisdom at work. Over time, cultural traditions, family habits, and societal pressures shape our relationship with food. Diets, with their restrictive rules, often fail to honor this inner wisdom, instead imposing external control.

Here, we focus on reconnecting you with that intuitive, healthy part of yourself. We peel away the layers—the habits, beliefs, and emotions—that have weighed you down for so long.

Start small: Pause before eating and ask yourself, "What am I really hungry for?" Often, it's not food but comfort, connection, or calm.

Peeling Back the Layers

Think of an onion. To get to its core, you must peel back the outer layers. This program works the same way:

- Evoke: First, we build a foundation of confidence and self-belief by exploring your history and uncovering the root causes of your weight struggles.

- Embrace: Next, we validate your experiences and accept all parts of you—the good, the bad, and the complicated. By embracing your whole self, you create space for healing and growth.

- Evolve: Finally, we release the old patterns, thoughts, and habits that no longer serve you, allowing the healthiest, most vibrant version of yourself to emerge.

Think of this week as a time to reflect: What patterns have been holding you back? Are they linked to comfort, stress, or even old family traditions?

Affirmation: *"I am ready to evoke what was, embrace what is, and evolve into what will be. My history matters, but it does not define me. I am here to create a new reality for myself - because I matter. From this day forward, every day in every way, I feel better than yesterday, yet not as good as tomorrow. And so it is!"*

Magda's Story: Finding the Sweetness in Life

Magda adored donuts. Every Friday, she'd treat herself to one at work. But as we explored her patterns, she realized donuts weren't just a snack—they were a connection to her grandfather, who always brought her donuts as a child.

Through our sessions, Magda began to honor the sweet memories without relying on sugary treats. She started journaling about her grandfather's stories and occasionally indulged in a donut—not out of habit but as a mindful choice. Within weeks, she found sweetness in her life by connecting with loved ones and baking healthy snacks with her kids.

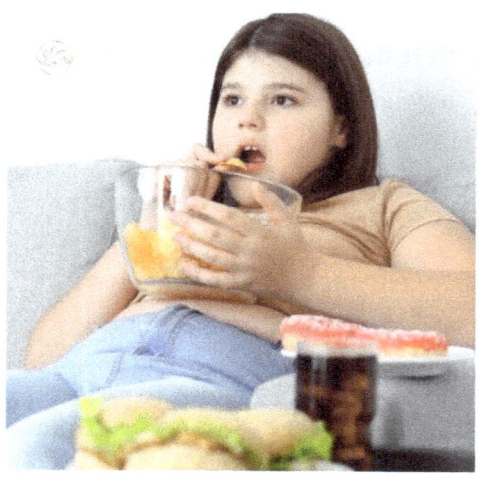

Discovering Your Patterns

Let me begin by sharing Magda's story. Magda, a woman in her late 30s, felt imprisoned by a cycle of emotional eating. Stress at work, coupled with feelings of loneliness, sent her reaching for comfort food every evening.

She described the behavior as "automatic," a habit she felt powerless to break. When we began working together, Magda started to uncover the deeper roots of her habits—unresolved feelings of loneliness, inadequacy, anxiety, and childhood messages tied to food. To ignore what was happening in the house, she'd zone out watching TV and indulging in sweets.

She remembered her grandfather saying: "You are as sweet as this donut!" Through awareness and intentional action, she slowly rewrote her patterns, embracing her sweetness with healthier fruits and personality, and new behaviors that aligned with the life she truly wanted. She no longer needed to be as sweet as the donut, but who she was.

This week, it's your turn to uncover the patterns that have been silently guiding your life.

Your Journey Starts Here

Every step you take, no matter how small, brings you closer to the life you deserve. Keep stepping forward, one choice at a time.

Quote of the Week:

"It's not what you weigh that matters—it's shedding and letting go of what's been weighing you down." ~ Liza

Exercise: Recognizing Your Patterns

If you have reached this far, then that alone is a testament to your strength and willingness to evolve.

Take a few minutes to reflect:

1. **When do I usually overeat or make unhealthy food choices?**

   - Is it after a stressful day or during celebrations?

2. **What emotions or triggers lead me to eat?**

   - Boredom, loneliness, or the need for comfort?

3. **What memories or stories are tied to my favorite foods?**

   - Are they linked to family traditions, celebrations, or moments of comfort?

The "layers" you've carried might include:

- Emotional eating or stress-eating.

- Cravings for unhealthy foods.

- Sedentary habits or lack of exercise.

- Toxic physical and emotional environments.

- Misunderstandings about nutrition.

- A negative self-image.

These aren't personal failures—they're patterns and responses that developed over time. And here's the truth: They're not permanent. You have the power to peel them away and reveal the healthy, vibrant person within.

Write your answers in your journal. Be honest and kind with yourself—it's all part of the process.

The Role of Triggers

Triggers are like sneaky ninjas—silent until they strike. Whether it's your boss's "urgent" email or the sound of a bag of chips opening, recognizing these moments is the first step to outsmarting them.

Pro tip: Next time a trigger strikes, pause. Take a deep breath, swallow your saliva, and ask yourself, "Am I truly hungry, or do I need something else right now?" Replace the automatic response with a glass of water and an empowering new choice.

Affirmations and Self-Talk

Positive affirmations help reframe your mindset and create new, empowering patterns. Catch yourself saying, "I can't do this"? Replace it with, "I am capable of creating positive change."

Try these affirmations:

- "I honor my body and its needs."
- "I choose nourishing foods that support my health."
- "I am in control of my choices."

We're Cheering You On

No single method or plan is a "magic bullet." True transformation requires intention, consistency, and support— and that's where we come in. You are not alone on this journey. We're here to hold you accountable and cheer you on every step of the way.

This is your time to Stand Up, let go of what's been weighing you down, and embrace the freedom, health, and joy that await you.

Weekly Action Steps

1. **Keep a Food Journal:** Write down not just what you eat but how you feel before and after. Notice patterns.

2. **Pause Before Eating:** Ask, "Am I physically hungry, or do I need to feed a need, or something else?"

3. **Celebrate Small Wins:** Each time you make a mindful choice, acknowledge it. Growth happens one step at a time.

Reflection: Building Awareness

As you move through this week, embrace curiosity over judgment. Discovering your patterns isn't about finding fault— it's about understanding yourself better. Each insight is a step toward creating the life you truly desire.

Your "Why" Revisited

Let's reconnect with the "why" you discovered last week. Why are you here? Why do you want to release old patterns and create a lighter, freer life?

Ie: *"I'm doing this to feel confident when I walk into a room. I want to show my daughter that self-love is powerful and possible at any age."*

Your "why" is your guiding star—a reminder of what you're striving for and the life you're creating. It's not just a thought; it's your anchor, your motivation, and your source of strength when the journey feels challenging. Take a moment to write your "why" in clear, powerful, and personal words. Once you've written it, make it visible. Here's how you can integrate it into your daily life:

- **Use Post-it Notes:** Write your "why" on several sticky notes and place them where you'll see them daily—your bathroom mirror, refrigerator, closet door, or dashboard.

- **Digital Reminders:** Set your "why" as the screensaver on your phone or computer, so it's the first thing you see when you start your day.

- **In Your Journal:** Write your "why" at the top of each page as a daily affirmation.

- **Create a Vision Board:** Include your "why" alongside images and words that inspire you, placing it in a spot where you can see it regularly.

Each morning, take a moment to read your "why" out loud. Let it sink in. Let it energize you. Let it remind you why you're making these changes—not for anyone else, but for yourself. Your "why" is your promise to yourself—one you are fully capable of keeping.

The 2-Step Process for Transformation

Nadine, one of my clients, once told me, "I thought I needed to change my body to feel happy, but I learned I had to start with my mind first." This insight is the core of the transformation process. Many people believe that dropping weight is all about diet and exercise, but the truth is deeper—it's about transforming from the inside out.

This process has two key steps: Awareness and Action.

Step 1: Awareness

Before any meaningful change can occur, you need to become aware of the patterns, beliefs, and emotions driving your current behaviors. Awareness is the spotlight that illuminates the shadows. Without it, you're navigating your journey blindfolded.

Ask Yourself: What am I holding on to?

Maybe it's an outdated belief like, "I've always been the 'big one' in the family." Or a memory of someone teasing you about your weight that still stings today.

Why do I make the choices I make?

For instance, are you grabbing junk food because it's convenient, or because it's comforting after a stressful day?

How does my body feel right now?

Tune in. Is there tension, heaviness, or discomfort? Your body holds onto emotions, and they often show up physically.

When you start to observe yourself without judgment, you create space for change.

Step 2: Action

Awareness alone won't transform your life. You need to pair it with intentional, consistent action. This doesn't mean overhauling everything overnight. Small, manageable steps taken daily lead to big results over time.

Start with these Actions:

Practice Mindful Eating: Take time to savor each bite. Notice the flavors, textures, and how your body feels as you eat. This simple practice helps you reconnect with your body's hunger and fullness signals.

Journal Daily: Write about your thoughts, feelings, and experiences. What patterns are you noticing? What small wins can you celebrate?

Make One Healthy Swap: Replace soda with water or swap out chips for fresh fruit. Start small; these tiny actions add up.

Lifestyle Changes: A Foundation for Lasting Transformation

Once you've built awareness and taken your first steps, it's time to lay the foundation for a healthier, more vibrant lifestyle. Remember, this isn't about perfection—it's about progress. You're not just changing what you do; you're transforming who you are.

1. Create a Supportive Environment

Your surroundings influence your habits. If your pantry is stocked with chips and cookies, it's easy to reach for them when cravings strike. Make your environment work for you.

Action Step: Clean out your kitchen. Stock it with nutritious, satisfying foods that fuel your body and align with your goals.

2. Move Your Body with Love

Exercise shouldn't feel like punishment. Instead, think of it as a celebration of what your body can do. Whether it's a brisk walk, dancing in your living room, or a yoga session, find movement you enjoy.

Action Step: Commit to moving your body for 20-30 minutes at least three times this week. Make it fun—play your favorite music or invite a friend to join you.

3. Cultivate a Growth Mindset

Your mindset shapes your reality. When challenges arise, how you perceive them determines your ability to overcome them.

Adopting a growth mindset means seeing obstacles as opportunities to learn and grow.

Action Step: The next time you face a setback, pause and reframe it. Instead of saying, "I failed," try, "This is a chance to learn and adjust."

4. Prioritize Sleep and Rest
Your body heals, restores, and regenerates during sleep. Lack of sleep can disrupt your hormones, increase cravings, and sap your energy.

Action Step: Set a bedtime routine. Aim for 7-8 hours of quality sleep each night. Create a calming ritual, like reading or meditating, to help you unwind.

5. Practice Gratitude Daily

Gratitude shifts one's focus from what one lacks to what one has. It's a simple yet powerful way to cultivate positivity and resilience.

Action Step: Write down three things you're grateful for each morning. Let this practice anchor your day in abundance.

A Reflection on Progress

As we close this week, let me remind you that transformation is a journey, not a destination. It's about showing up for yourself daily, even when it feels hard. It's about celebrating small wins and extending compassion to yourself when you stumble.

Here's a thought to carry with you: "The greatest wealth is health. But health isn't just physical—it's mental, emotional, and spiritual. When you nurture all parts of yourself, you unlock the life you deserve."

Weekly Action Steps

Commit to Awareness: Reflect on the patterns and triggers you uncovered this week. Write about them in your journal.

Take One Action: Choose one healthy habit to start this week— mindful eating, drinking more water, or walking.

Revisit Your "Why": Place your "why" in a visible spot and read it daily. Let it ground and motivate you.

Practice Gratitude: Start each day with three things you're grateful for.

Be Kind to Yourself: Replace negative self-talk with affirmations. Speak to yourself as you would to a loved one.

By the end of this week, you'll notice subtle but powerful shifts within yourself. You're becoming more aware, intentional, and aligned with your goals. Keep going—you're stronger than you think, and the best is yet to come.

Let's continue this journey together in Week Three when we'll explore how to embrace and honor your unique body, mind, and spirit.

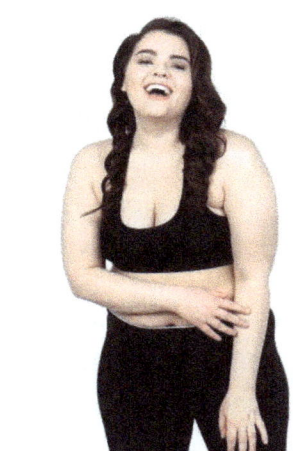

WEEK THREE - Embrace and Honor Your Unique Self

Welcome to Week Three

Congratulations on making it to Week Three! You've begun a transformative process by evoking your past and uncovering patterns that no longer serve you. This week, we shift the focus to embracing and honoring the incredible individual you are—body, mind, and spirit.

Take a deep breath and place your hand on your heart. Remind yourself: this journey isn't about perfection; it's about progress, self-compassion, and creating a life that feels aligned with your true essence. Each step you take is a celebration of your courage and commitment.

The Power of Embracing Yourself

Imagine Camille, a woman in her early 60s, who had spent years battling self-criticism. Each time she stood in front of the mirror, her focus was on what she thought was "wrong." She'd sigh, "My arms are too flabby," or, "My stomach will never look the way it used to." These harsh thoughts left her drained and stuck in a cycle of negativity.

When Camille began this journey, she discovered that her body was not the enemy—it was her greatest ally. She learned to honor her body for its strength, its resilience, and the stories it carried. As Camille shifted her focus to celebrating what her body could do instead of what it couldn't, she found a newfound sense of peace and appreciation.

Like Camille, you have the power to change the way you see yourself. Instead of striving for an unrealistic ideal, this week is about embracing your unique beauty and celebrating the body, mind, and spirit that make you - *you*.

Honoring Your Body

Your body is a miracle. It adapts, heals, and carries you through life's challenges. Yet, it's easy to focus on what we perceive as flaws instead of celebrating its wonders.

Your body carries you through life, adapts to challenges, and supports you in ways you may not even realize. Yet, how often do you criticize it instead of appreciating it?

Think of the language you use when talking about your body. Are your words kind, or are they harsh? Remember, your body hears everything you say. Instead of saying, "I hate my thighs," try, "I'm grateful for my legs—they carry me everywhere I go."

Journaling Prompt: A Love Letter to Your Body

Take 10 minutes to write a love letter to your body. Start with "Dear Body," and express gratitude for all it does for you. Apologize for any unkind words or neglect and commit to treating it with kindness and care moving forward.

How Does Your Belly Feel?

Take a moment to pause and check in with your body. How does your belly feel right now? Is it tight, bloated, or heavy? Or maybe squishy, soft, or just there? These physical sensations are your body's way of speaking to you, but beneath them lies an emotional layer.

Your belly carries more than food; it holds emotions like anxiety, loneliness, joy, and even despair. This isn't just metaphorical—your belly is the core of your life force, and it responds directly to your mental and emotional state. It's no surprise that when you feel stressed, nervous, or sad, your stomach often reacts. The gut is sometimes called your "second brain" because of its deep connection to your emotions through the gut-brain axis.

Now we dive into the emotions your belly might be carrying and how they impact your journey to drop weight.

Fat Feeling #1: Loneliness

Because It Messes Up Your Hunger Hormones

Loneliness can feel like an emptiness that food often seems to fill. But the truth is, loneliness does more than just encourage emotional eating—it affects your hormones. Studies have shown that people who feel lonely experience higher levels of ghrelin, a hunger hormone. This means you feel hungrier more often, even after eating, driving you to consume more calories than your body needs.

Break the Mood: Step away from your screen. Social media might seem like a cure for loneliness, but it often intensifies the feeling of disconnection. Instead, take a walk or join a group that shares your interests. Whether it's yoga, book clubs, or simply meeting a friend for tea, connecting face-to-face can reduce those hunger cues.

Fat Feeling #2: Deprivation

Because It Manifests as Hunger

Deprivation isn't just about food—it's about the areas of your life where you feel you're lacking. Whether it's love, adventure, or validation, deprivation can show up as cravings for comfort foods. Your brain is wired to view forbidden things as rewards, which is why dieting often backfires. The more you tell yourself you "can't" have something, the more you want it.

Break the Mood: Allow yourself small indulgences.

Fat Feeling #3: Stress

Because It Triggers Fat Storage

Stress wreaks havoc on your body in ways you might not even realize. When you're stressed, your body releases adrenaline to prepare for a fight-or-flight response. While this was useful when we had to outrun predators, today's stresses—deadlines, traffic, bills—don't require that physical energy. Unused adrenaline leads to the release of cortisol, another hormone that tells your body to store fat, particularly in the belly region.

Break the Mood: Laughter is one of the simplest and most effective ways to reduce stress. Watch a funny movie, share a joke with a friend, or find a moment to play with your kids or pets. Laughter helps lower cortisol levels and reminds your body to relax.

Fat Feeling #4: Boredom

Because It Confuses Your Brain

Boredom often tricks your brain into thinking you're hungry. Without purposeful engagement, your mind seeks stimulation, and food becomes an easy fix. Boredom-induced eating is a double-edged sword because not only do you eat more, but you also make poorer food choices.

Break the Mood: Instead of seeking entertainment, look for purpose. Volunteer, learn a new skill, or challenge yourself with a creative project. Purposeful activity not only distracts you from food but also nourishes your soul.

Fat Feeling #5: Anxiety

Because It Leads to Disordered Eating

Anxiety keeps your body in a constant state of stress, making it one of the most significant triggers for weight gain. Research shows that anxiety often precedes disordered eating, creating a cycle that's difficult to break. The constant worry and fear fuel cravings for quick comfort, usually in the form of sugary, fatty foods.

Break the Mood: Combine exercise with nature. A brisk walk in the park or a bike ride through the countryside can significantly reduce anxiety. Physical activity releases endorphins, while nature soothes your nervous system, creating a powerful combination for calming your mind.

Fat Feeling #6: Coupled Bliss

Because It Encourages Shared Habits

Being in a loving relationship is wonderful, but it can also lead to shared unhealthy habits. Regular meals together, larger portions, and less emphasis on staying active can cause both partners to gain weight over time. Studies show that weight gain often increases in the comfort of a relationship, while weight loss can accompany a breakup.

Break the Mood: Turn your relationship into a support system for healthy habits. Eat nutritious meals together, go for walks. Weight loss can be a shared goal that strengthens your bond while improving your health.

Your Core: A Source of Wisdom

Your belly isn't just a physical space; it's your core, the center of your being. When you tune in to what your body is telling you, you gain insight into your emotional and physical health. Your belly holds the stories of your life—the joys, pains, the lessons. By listening to it, you can begin to release the heaviness, both literal and metaphorical, that no longer serves you.

Weekly Action Steps

1. Tune Into Your Emotions: Take a moment each day to ask, "How do I feel right now?" Write down your answers and notice any patterns between your emotions and your cravings.
2. Shift the Narrative: When you feel a strong craving or impulse, pause and ask, "What am I needing?" Replace the urge to eat with an action that fulfills the underlying need—call a friend, take a walk, or practice deep breathing.
3. Start Gratitude Practice: Each night, list three things about your body that you're grateful for. This simple practice builds a positive relationship with your physical self.
4. Choose One Area to Improve: Whether it's reducing stress, managing boredom, or connecting with others, commit to making one change this week.

Quote to Inspire

"Your body hears everything your mind says. Speak love, kindness, and healing." ~ Unknown

Mind Matters: Nurturing the Core of Your Being

Think back to your childhood. Can you recall moments when you were taken somewhere you dreaded—perhaps a tedious errand or a visit to a distant relative? Contrast that with the times you were taken to a park, the fair, or your favorite place. Remember how boundless your energy felt and how alive you were?

These memories reflect the powerful influence of emotions on our energy and bodies. Our bodies are physical representations of our feelings, expressing the emotions we've carried, suppressed, or processed. The connection between our mind and body shapes our well-being on every level.

As Sir William Osler, the "father of psychosomatic medicine," wisely said: *"The hurt that does not find its expression through tears may cause other organs to weep."*

Unprocessed emotions don't simply disappear. They settle into our bodies, influencing how we feel, function, and heal.

The Power of Processing Loss and Hurt

Loss is a natural part of life. It often manifests as hurt in the present, transforms into anger when tied to the past, and becomes fear when projected into the future. Each of these emotions impacts our health and shapes our ability to live freely.

Animals instinctively express emotions like fear or anger to create boundaries. Humans, however, often suppress these feelings, bottling up anger, denying fears, and smiling through pain. Over time, this emotional suppression weighs us down—physically, mentally, and emotionally.

Take a moment to reflect:

- How did your parents handle emotions when you were a child?

- Were you encouraged or discouraged from expressing your feelings?

- Is there a memory or person from your childhood that still evokes strong emotions today?

Honest reflection can bring clarity, helping you understand how these patterns influence your relationship with yourself now.

The Weight of Family Expectations

For many, weight struggles are intertwined with family dynamics. Perhaps some of your loved ones share similar habits, and your decision to change feels like an act of betrayal. You might hear:

- "Why are you trying to be different from us?"

- "Are you saying there's something wrong with how we live?"

- "Do you think you're better than us?"

Does any of this resonate? Fear of alienating loved ones can hold you back from pursuing your goals. But remember this isn't about rejecting your family—it's about honoring yourself.

Ask yourself:

- Whose voice have you been afraid to stand up to?

- What inner voice stops you from breaking free?

Your journey is yours alone. By honoring your needs, you inspire others to reflect on their own.

The Connection Between Mind and Body

The term "psychosomatic" is often misunderstood. It doesn't mean "all in your head." Instead, it reflects the undeniable connection between the mind and body. What we hold in our minds manifests in our bodies. Think of common phrases like:

- *"Sick with worry"*
- *"Scared stiff"*
- *"A pain in the neck"*

These expressions aren't just metaphors—they reflect real, physical responses to emotional states. Chronic stress, fatigue, and unresolved emotions take a toll on our bodies, creating patterns of tension, pain, and even illness.

Reclaiming Your Power

True healing begins when you stop seeking approval outside yourself and turn inward. It means trusting your intuition, honoring your needs, and taking responsibility for your happiness.

Reflect on these questions:

- What do you see when you look in the mirror?

- When did you feel like you lost control of your weight?

- Are there parts of your body you've struggled to accept?

- What do you admire about others, and how can you nurture those qualities in yourself?

Your answers hold the key to understanding your relationship with your body and mind.

Weekly Action Steps

Reflect on Your Emotional Landscape: Use a journal to explore the questions above. Let your answers reveal the patterns shaping your habits. Identify a Voice to Stand Up To: Whether it's an external voice or your inner critic, challenge it with compassion and strength.

Reconnect with Your Core: Spend 5 minutes daily with your hands on your belly, breathing deeply, and asking, "What do I need right now?"

Practice Affirmations: Start with "I honor my emotions and listen to my body's wisdom."

Take One Loving Action: Prepare a nourishing meal, go for a walk, or say "no" to something that doesn't serve you.

Affirmations for Embracing Yourself

Use these affirmations daily to reinforce positive self-talk:

- "I honor and cherish my body."
- "I am grateful for the strength and beauty within me."
- "Every part of me tells a story, and I embrace it with love."

Reflection:

This week, take time to notice moments when you feel gratitude for your body. Maybe it's when you climb a set of stairs, hold a loved one close, or take a calming breath. Celebrate these moments—they are proof of your strength and resilience.

Quote to Inspire

"You carry so much love in your heart.
Give some to yourself." ~ R.Z.

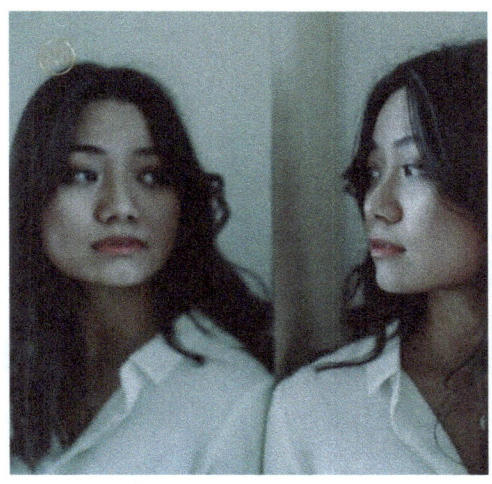

The Power of Mirror Work: Seeing and Embracing Your True Self

When was the last time you truly looked at yourself in the mirror—not to check your hair, apply makeup, or critique your appearance, but to *see* yourself? For many, the answer might be "never." We often use the mirror as a tool to focus on what's wrong or what we wish to fix. Yet, the mirror has the potential to be one of the most profound instruments of self-healing, self-acceptance, and transformation.

Mirrorwork goes beyond surface-level gazing. It's about connecting deeply with the person staring back at you—acknowledging, appreciating, and embracing all that you are. For some, this can feel intimidating or even painful. After all, the mirror doesn't just reflect our physical selves; it reflects our inner emotions, fears, and insecurities. But it also holds the potential to reflect love, strength, and courage.

Why Mirror Work Matters

Most people fall into two camps when it comes to mirrors: those who avoid them altogether and those who spend too much time critiquing themselves in them. Both approaches can disconnect us from our true selves. Mirror work invites us to shift from using the mirror as a tool of judgment to a space of self-compassion and acknowledgment.

The mirror becomes a witness to your journey—a silent companion as you learn to meet yourself where you are, with love and acceptance. This practice can be life-changing because it forces you to confront your thoughts, beliefs, and emotions head-on. It creates a space where you can affirm your worth, challenge negative self-talk, and build a deeper relationship with yourself.

How to Begin Mirror Work

Mirror work is simple in practice but profound in impact. Here's how to start:

1. Find a Quiet Moment: Stand in front of a mirror where you won't be interrupted. It doesn't need to be a full-length mirror—a small one will do if you can see your face.

2. Look into Your Own Eyes: This might feel awkward at first, but stay with it. Imagine looking beyond the surface, beyond your reflection, and into your soul. What do you see? What do you feel?

3. Speak to Yourself with Love: Say three things you appreciate about yourself. These can be physical traits, accomplishments, or qualities you admire. Start small if needed.

For example:
- "I'm proud of myself for showing up today."
- "I love my laugh; it brings joy to others."
- "I appreciate my resilience; I've overcome so much."

4. **Repeat Daily:** Commit to this practice for at least 21 days. Over time, notice how it feels. At first, it might feel forced or uncomfortable. You may even want to look away. That's okay—stick with it. With time, the discomfort fades, replaced by a growing sense of self-acceptance and love.

The Depth of Mirror Work

Mirror work isn't just an affirmation practice; it's an act of courage. It requires vulnerability to face yourself fully, without filters or distractions. It's a way of saying to yourself: *I see you. I hear you. You matter.*

Some people find that emotions rise to the surface during this practice—tears, frustration, or even resistance. These emotions are not barriers; they are breakthroughs. They are signs that you are peeling back layers of self-judgment and moving toward self-compassion.

Consider this: When we look in the mirror with intention, we start to rewrite the narrative we've been telling ourselves for years. Instead of focusing on flaws, we begin to see beauty. Instead of critiquing imperfections, we start acknowledging our worth.

A Client's Journey with Mirror Work

Katherine, a client of mine, once told me she avoided mirrors for years. She couldn't bear to look at herself without immediately falling into a spiral of self-criticism. When I introduced her to mirror work, she was skeptical. But she committed to it, starting with just one affirmation a day: *"I'm proud of myself for trying."*

At first, she said it felt hollow, like she was lying to herself. But as the days turned into weeks, something shifted. She began to feel the words instead of just saying them. She started noticing her strength, her beauty, and her worth. By the end of the program, Katherine told me, *"I don't just see my reflection anymore. I see someone I love."*

Why Mirror Work Can Transform Your Journey

Your reflection is more than what you see on the surface. It's a gateway to your inner world. Mirror work aligns perfectly with the principles of Evoking, Embracing, and Evolving:

- Evoke: Bring to light the stories, beliefs, and emotions you've held about yourself. Confront them with honesty.
- Embrace: Accept yourself fully, imperfections and all. Meet yourself with kindness, just as you would a dear friend.
- Evolve: Use this practice as a foundation to build self-love, confidence, and a deeper connection with who you are.

Weekly Mirror Work Challenge

1. **Start Small:** Begin each morning with one positive affirmation in the mirror. Look yourself in the eyes and say, *"I am worthy of love and care."*
2. **Add Layers:** As you grow more comfortable, expand your affirmations to include qualities you admire about yourself or goals you are working toward.
3. **Journal the Journey:** After each session, jot down how you feel. Are you noticing shifts in your self-talk? Are there emotions coming up that surprise you?
4. **Celebrate Progress:** At the end of the week, reflect on your growth. What have you learned about yourself? What are you proud of?

Quote to Inspire

"You've been criticizing yourself for years, and it hasn't worked. Try approving of yourself and see what happens." ~ Louise Hay

Connecting with Your Spirit-Beyond the Body

Who you are is so much more than what you see in the mirror.

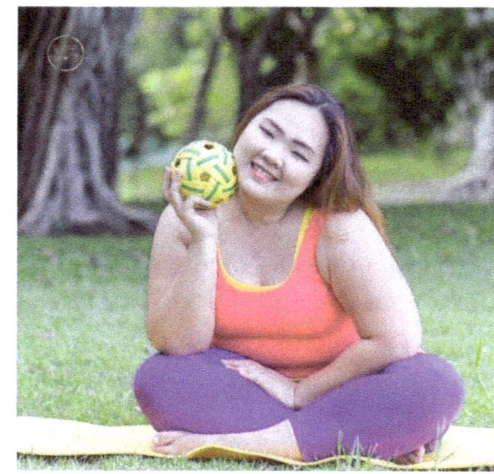

Your body is your home, but it is not your identity. As Dr. Wayne Dyer so eloquently said,

"We are not human beings having a spiritual experience; we are spiritual beings having a human experience."

Take that in.
You are a soul—eternal, wise, powerful—temporarily living in this physical form.
Your shape, size, weight, or age does not define you. They are part of your earthly journey, but not the whole of who you are.

The journey to wellness, therefore, is not just about reshaping your body; it's about reconnecting with the essence of your spirit. That part of you that dreams without limits, that believes in magic, and that longs to feel joy for no reason at all.

When you begin to connect within beyond the flesh, beyond expectations, you awaken a deeper motivation for change. You no longer chase weight loss to "look better" for others. You begin to care for your body because your spirit deserves a safe, healthy, and vibrant place to live.

This is the true shift—from punishment to partnership.
From shame to sacredness.
From fixing your body to honoring your being.

Honoring Your Spirit

Your spirit is the source of your intuition, creativity, love, and resilience.
It's the quiet voice that says *keep going,* even when your mind is tired.
It's the feeling of peace when you're aligned, and the nudge of discomfort when you're not.

To honor your spirit is to allow joy.
To invite stillness.
To move from a deeper why.

Try This: Daily Joy Practice

Each day, commit to one small act that lights you up. It doesn't have to be grand—it just needs to feel good.

- Dance to your favorite song.
- Watch the sunset with full attention.
- Speak kindly to yourself in the mirror.
- Savor a warm cup of tea.
- Hug your child a little longer.
  These moments remind you: *I am alive. I am worthy. I am more than this body.*

Weekly Action Steps

1. Practice Mirror Work
   Each morning or evening, stand before your reflection.
   Look into your eyes. Say something loving—something
   true. Remind yourself: *This body has carried me through
   everything. I choose to honor it.*

2. Write a Love Letter to Your Body
   Grab your journal and write to your body as if it were a
   dear friend. Acknowledge its strength, its sacrifices, and
   its ability to keep showing up, even when you've been
   unkind. Gratitude opens the door to healing.

3. Shift Your Language
   Notice the way you speak about yourself—out loud and
   in your thoughts. Would you say those things to
   someone you love? If not, shift it. Choose softer, kinder,
   more empowering words.

4. Prioritize Joy
   Schedule it. Don't wait for the perfect moment—create
   one. Joy is not frivolous—it is fuel for the soul.

5. Revisit Your "Why"
   Keep your motivation visible. Whether it's a note on
   your mirror or a reminder on your phone, reconnect
   daily with *why* you began this journey. Your "why" is
   your anchor when the waves of doubt try to pull you
   back.

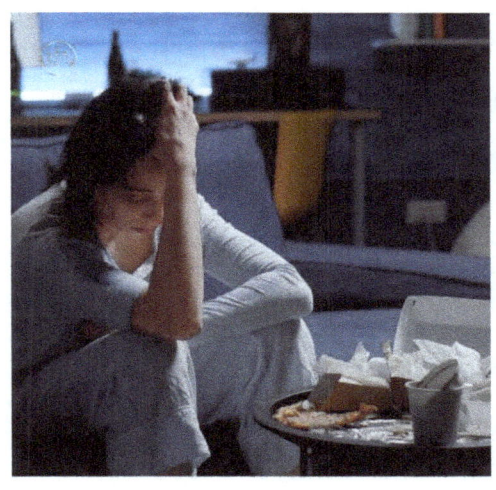

WEEK FOUR - Why Do You Eat the Way You Do?

By now, you've begun uncovering your patterns, embracing self-compassion, and connecting with your "why." This week, we shift our focus to nourishment, not just through food but through thoughts, actions, and habits that uplift and support your body and mind.

Your body is your home—a sacred space that houses your spirit, dreams, and desires. Nourishing is about more than just food; it's about listening to its needs, treating it with kindness, and cultivating a harmonious relationship between your physical self and your inner world.

Why Do I Overeat—Do I Know?

We live in a society driven by instant gratification. Reality TV, online gambling, and countless quick-fix solutions are everywhere, and food is no exception. It's easy to reach for a snack, not because we're hungry, but because we crave comfort, escape, or a momentary reward. Over time, this has led to patterns of overeating and an epidemic of disconnection from our own bodies.

Let me ask you this: Why do you eat?

For many, the reasons go beyond hunger. You might say:

- "Because I love food."

- "It makes me feel better."

- "I'm bored, angry, stressed, or anxious."

- "I feel lonely or overwhelmed."

If any of these resonate, you're not alone. Overeating is rarely about hunger—it's about emotions, habits, and subconscious patterns that were often set long ago.

The Subconscious Patterns Behind Overeating

Have you ever caught yourself reaching for snacks when you weren't hungry? Next time it happens, pause and ask yourself: "What am I feeling right now?" Chances are, it's not physical hunger but an emotion—stress, boredom, sadness, or even celebration—that's driving the urge.

Think back to your childhood. Were you given candy to stop crying or rewarded with dessert for good behavior? Were you told to "clean your plate" because others were starving? These early messages often shape subconscious patterns, linking food to comfort, reward, or obligation. Over time, eating becomes less about fueling your body and more about soothing your emotions.

Camille's Story: Listening to Her Body

Remember Camille? Well, Camille came to me feeling trapped. She had been dieting for years, trying every new fad and obsessing over the scale, but nothing seemed to work. Despite her relentless efforts, she felt disconnected from her body. "I don't even know what my body needs anymore," she confessed during our first session. She had a goal of losing 10-15 pounds, but as we worked together, her journey turned into something much deeper.

Through our sessions, Camille began to uncover layers of self-doubt, shame, guilt, and even resentment toward herself. These emotions, buried for decades, were tied not just to her eating habits but also to her sense of self-worth. Slowly, we peeled back the negative patterns that had weighed her down, not just physically but emotionally.

As Camille began to shed these layers, she dropped 32 pounds—not because she starved herself or followed a rigid plan, but because she started to truly care for herself. She also made a courageous decision: after 35 years in a toxic and abusive marriage, Camille chose to separate. While she wasn't ready for divorce, she began reclaiming her life by taking tai chi classes, swimming, and exploring art. For the first time in years, she felt lighter—not just in her body but in her spirit.

Camille's story isn't about perfection. It's about transformation, courage, and partnership with oneself. She stopped fighting her body and started listening to it. She began nourishing it with food, movement, and self-love, regaining the sense of joy and vitality she had lost.

This week, I invite you to embark on a similar journey—not just of weight loss but of reconnection. Together, let's uncover the deeper reasons behind your eating habits and create a foundation of respect, nourishment, and self-care.

What Happens When You Ignore Your Feelings?

Pushing down your emotions doesn't make them disappear. Instead, they tend to resurface in unexpected ways. For many, they show up as emotional eating. The cookie jar becomes a source of comfort, the fridge a way to cope. But food can only distract you temporarily—it doesn't address the underlying emotions.

When you eat to avoid your feelings, you disconnect from yourself. Over time, this disconnection becomes a habit, and the cycle of emotional eating takes hold. You feel guilty for eating, and that guilt leads to more eating. It's a frustrating and exhausting loop—but it's not unbreakable.

The First Step to Freedom: Awareness

Breaking the cycle of emotional eating begins with awareness. Start by asking yourself:

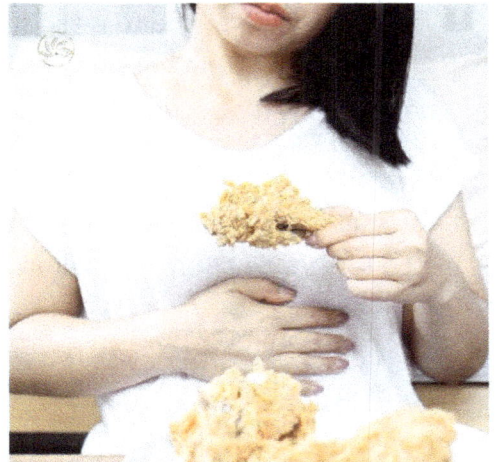

- What triggers my urge to eat?

- What emotions am I feeling before I reach for food?

- What am I truly craving—comfort, connection, relief?

The answers may not come easily, and that's okay. This is a process of self-discovery, one that requires patience and compassion.

Action Steps: Breaking the Cycle

1. Pause Before You Eat: The next time you feel the urge to snack, take a deep breath. Ask yourself, "Am I truly hungry, or am I feeling something else?"

2. Journal Your Emotions: Keep a journal of your feelings and eating habits. Over time, patterns will emerge, giving you insight into your triggers.

3. Find Alternative Comforts: Instead of turning to food, try other forms of self-care—take a walk, call a friend, or practice deep breathing. Be Kind to Yourself: If you slip into old habits, stop beating yourself up.

4. **When you begin from within, everything else aligns.**

5. This week, I invite you to walk in grace, breathe in gratitude, and treat your body as the sacred vessel it is— not because it's perfect, but because *you* are.

6. Let's commit to listening to your body, your emotions, and the messages they're sending. Together, we'll take another step toward freedom and self-love.

Quote to Inspire:

"Food is not your enemy. It's a tool for nourishment, not a replacement for love, connection, or joy. The real work is within you."

WHEN

I eat when I am...	Yes	No	New Choice
Hungry	__	__	_____
Nervous	__	__	_____
Bored	__	__	_____
Stressed	__	__	_____
Hyperactive	__	__	_____
Happy	__	__	_____

I eat when I am...	Yes	No	New Choice
Sad	__	__	_____
Lonely	__	__	_____
Frustrated	__	__	_____
Anxious	__	__	_____
Afraid	__	__	_____

Don't know what else to do

	Yes	No	New Choice
	__	__	_____
Relationship problems	__	__	_____
Work problems	__	__	_____
Family problems	__	__	_____

WHERE

I overeat or snack...

	Yes	No	New Choice
While watching TV	__	__	_____
In front of the computer			
	__	__	_____
While reading	__	__	_____
During coffee breaks	__	__	_____
Between office/home	__	__	_____
At business lunches	__	__	_____
At social events	__	__	_____
In bed	__	__	_____

WHY

I treat myself to a snack or meal...

	Yes	No	New Choice
When I Feel Loved	__	__	_____
To Reward Myself	__	__	_____
Something to do	__	__	_____
A change in my activity	__	__	_____

I treat myself to a snack or meal...

	Yes	No	New Choice
To deal with something unpleasant			
	__	__	_____
To relax	__	__	_____
To feel more important			
	__	__	_____
To feel secure	__	__	_____
To generate sexual attention			
	__	__	_____
Reminds me of the good old days			
	__	__	_____

How did you feel responding to these questions?

Did you gain a new insight into your patterns?

Take a moment and write a few words about how you feel right now.

_____

_____

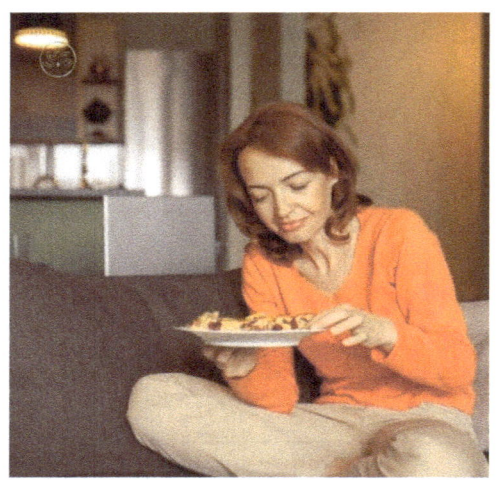

WEEK FIVE - Using Food as Protection

Welcome to Week Five!

By now, you've uncovered patterns, embraced truths about yourself, and begun reconnecting with your body. This week, we dive into the question that lies at the heart of emotional eating: **What are you craving?**

Spoiler alert: It's rarely about the food.

Meet Suzy: A Sweet Story of Transformation

Suzy had an unwavering love for chocolate chip cookies. Every evening, like clockwork, she'd curl up on her couch with a plate of cookies and a cup of tea. "It's my little ritual," she told me during our first session. Suzy swore she couldn't imagine life without those cookies. But as we worked together in hypnotherapy, we discovered that her nightly cookie ritual wasn't just about enjoying a sweet treat—it was about comfort, connection, and something far deeper.

Through our sessions, Suzy traced her love for cookies back to her childhood. Her grandmother, a warm, nurturing presence in her life, always had cookies waiting when Suzy came to visit. They'd sit together at the kitchen table—her grandma with a book in hand, reading aloud, while little Suzy nibbled on those freshly baked cookies. To Suzy, those moments were pure magic—filled with love, warmth, and safety.

But as an adult, Suzy's cookie habit wasn't giving her the same satisfaction. Instead, it had become a nightly reflex, a way to soothe herself after stressful days. Through hypnotherapy, Suzy uncovered this deep connection to her grandmother and realized what she truly craved wasn't the cookies themselves but the feelings they symbolized—love, comfort, and the joy of storytelling.

With this newfound awareness, Suzy didn't have to "give up" her cookies. Instead, she replaced the habit with something meaningful: books. She began curling up with a novel instead of a plate of cookies, rediscovering her love for stories and the sense of connection they brought her. Suzy still enjoyed cookies occasionally, but they no longer held the same power. Now, she savored them without guilt, knowing her real craving wasn't for the cookies but for the sense of warmth and care they once represented.

What about you? When you reach for that bag of chips or another slice of pizza, what are you truly hungry for? This week, let's dig deeper into the needs beneath your food choices and explore new ways to nourish your heart and mind.

"Nourishing yourself in a way that helps you blossom in the direction you want to go is attainable, and you are worth the effort." ~ Deborah Day

The Real Hunger: It's Not Always About Food

Food is an easy answer to emotional hunger because it's readily available, culturally acceptable, and comforting in the moment. But often, true hunger isn't physical—it's emotional or spiritual. Consider these common "hungers":

- **Comfort:** Do you use food to soothe stress or sadness?

- **Control:** When life feels chaotic, do you turn to food as the one thing you can manage?

- **Connection:** Are you eating to fill a void of loneliness or disconnection?

- **Celebration:** Do you associate food with joy and use it to create a sense of happiness?

Exercise: Uncovering Your True Cravings

This week, before you eat, take a moment to pause and reflect. Ask yourself these questions:

1. **Am I physically hungry, or is this an emotional craving?**

   o Check in with your body. Are you feeling hunger pangs, or is your desire for food coming from somewhere else?

2. **What am I feeling right now?**

   o Are you stressed, bored, lonely, or happy? Identifying your emotions is the first step to understanding your cravings.

3. **What do I truly need?**

    o   If it's not food, what could meet your needs?
        A hug? A break? Some fun or relaxation?

Write your answers in your journal. Over time, you'll start to
notice patterns, just like Suzy did.

Humor Break: A Lighthearted Look at Cravings

Here's a little humor to keep things light:

*"I'm not hungry, I'm bored. And I know this because I just ate an
entire meal, and now I'm eyeing the chips like they owe me
money."*

Sound familiar? Cravings can feel ridiculous at times, but
they're also deeply human. It's okay to laugh at yourself—it's
part of the process.

Replacing Food with Fulfillment

Once you've identified what you're craving, it's time to find
non-food ways to meet your needs. Here are some ideas:

*   **For Comfort:** Wrap yourself in a cozy blanket, take a
    warm bath, or listen to soothing music.

*   **For Control:** Organize a small space in your home, like a
    drawer or closet. Accomplishing something tangible can
    restore a sense of balance.

*   **For Connection:** Call a friend, join a class, or spend time
    with loved ones.

- **For Celebration:** Dance to your favorite song, treat yourself to a non-food reward, or write down what you're grateful for.

Weekly Action Steps

1. **Pause Before Eating:** Practice reflection exercises before each meal or snack. Ask yourself, "What am I craving?"

2. **Journal Your Cravings:** Keep a record of your emotions and needs throughout the week. Note the moments when you felt tempted to eat and what you discovered.

3. **Choose Non-Food Comforts:** Make a list of activities or practices that bring you joy and comfort and turn to them when cravings strike.

4. **Celebrate Your Wins:** Every time you pause, reflect, or choose a non-food way to meet your needs, acknowledge yourself. Progress deserves celebration!

Quote to Reflect On

"If hunger isn't the problem, food isn't the solution." ~ Unknown

This quote is a reminder to pause and look deeper. When you identify your true hunger and meet it with kindness, you'll find that food becomes nourishment, not a crutch.

Who Do I Want to Become?

This is your time to dream, to imagine, and to step into the version of yourself that you know you are capable of becoming.

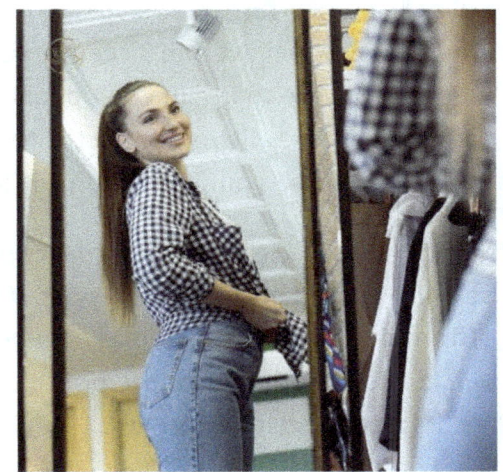

This exercise is not just about physical transformation—it's about stepping into the life, energy, and confidence that aligns with your vision.

Step 1: Ask

Take a moment to visualize your ideal self. What does she look like? How does she move through the world? Picture her in vivid detail—the sparkle in her eyes, the way she carries herself, the confidence radiating from her.

If you have photos of yourself at a weight or time when you felt vibrant and aligned, bring them out. Look at them often. If you don't, find images that represent the version of yourself you aspire to. Place these pictures where you'll see them daily—on your mirror, refrigerator, or as your phone's screensaver. Let them remind you of who you are becoming.

Step 2: Believe

Belief is a powerful force. To become the person you envision, you must first believe she already exists within you. Imagine what it feels like to live in your ideal body. How does it feel to wear clothes that fit you perfectly, to move freely, and to feel energized? Close your eyes and truly feel it.

Write out your ideal weight or description of your healthiest self and place it somewhere visible. If you use a scale, put this affirmation over the readout: *"I am becoming the healthiest version of myself."* Or choose not to weigh yourself at all and focus instead on how you feel.

Stop buying clothes that fit your current size as a way of settling. Instead, invest in pieces that reflect the person you're stepping into. Have faith that your vision is on its way to becoming your reality.

Think of this process as placing an order with the universe's catalog. You choose the version of yourself you want to embody, place the order, and trust it's being delivered. Your role is to stay aligned with that vision through your thoughts, words, and actions.

Silencing the Negative Chatter

Negative self-talk can be one of the biggest roadblocks on your journey to transformation. But here's the truth: *You are not your negative thoughts.* They are just old stories and patterns you've carried, and it's time to let them go.

Turn Down the Volume

Bring to mind the negative chatter that holds you back. Maybe it's a voice telling you, "You'll never change," or "Why bother trying again?" Whose voice, is it? Is it truly yours, or does it belong to someone else—a parent, a teacher, a peer?

Now imagine turning that voice into something absurd. Picture it as a cartoon character—Daffy Duck, Bugs Bunny, or even a Teletubby. Hear those negative words being delivered in a silly, exaggerated voice. What happens to their power? They lose it. They become laughable. They no longer have control over you.

Replace the Chatter

Your next step is to replace those negative thoughts with empowering ones. Monitor your thoughts throughout the day. When you catch yourself slipping into negativity, pause and redirect. Here's a simple chart to help you reframe your inner dialogue:

Negative Thought	Positive Replacement
"I'll never lose weight."	"I am making progress every day."
"I can't resist junk food."	"I choose foods that nourish me."
"I'm not good enough."	"I am worthy of love and care."

Fill out this chart with your thoughts and replacements. Refer to it daily until positive self-talk becomes second nature.

The Power of Words and Imagination

Your subconscious mind is always listening—and it takes your words and thoughts as direct instructions. When you speak with fear, doubt, or criticism, your subconscious works to fulfill that reality, even if it's not what you consciously want. The same is true when you speak with love, clarity, and belief. Every word you say and every image you hold in your mind shapes how your body responds, how you feel, and how you behave. If you constantly say, *"I can't lose weight,"* your subconscious accepts that as truth and creates resistance.

But when you affirm, *"I am becoming healthier every day,"* your subconscious begins to align with that vision. What you imagine, feel, and speak becomes the blueprint your body and mind work to build

A Quote to Inspire You

"Whether you think you can, or you think you can't—you're right." ~ Henry Ford

Your thoughts shape your reality. Choose ones that uplift, inspire, and align with the person you're becoming. Remember, you are in control of your narrative. Let this week be the beginning of a kinder, more empowering dialogue with yourself.

You've got this!

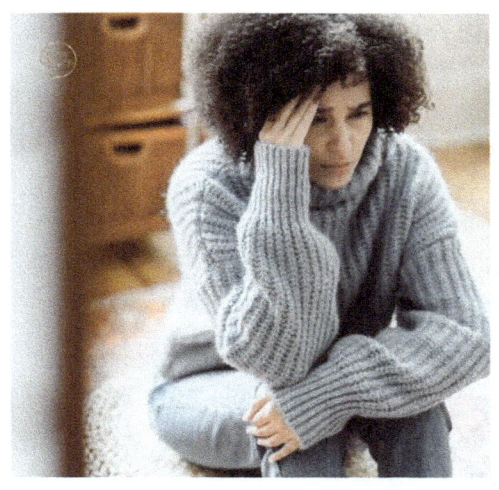

WEEK SIX - What Have I Been Avoiding?

In Week 4, you were introduced to Camille, a woman who had spent years dieting and feeling disconnected from her body. Through her journey, Camille discovered that her struggles weren't just about weight—they were tied to unspoken fears, limiting beliefs, and emotions she had avoided for decades. As she worked through the program, she began shedding more than her physical weight. Camille released toxic emotions, outdated beliefs, and even stepped away from a relationship that had kept her from living fully. Her transformation wasn't just physical—it was a reclaiming of her power.

This week, we'll dive deeper into what you might be avoiding. Often, the weight we carry isn't just on our bodies—it's in our hearts and minds. Camille's story teaches us that avoidance isn't a sign of weakness—it's a response to unprocessed feelings. But once you face those emotions, you can unlock a powerful shift toward freedom and self-empowerment.

Take a moment to pause and reflect:

What have I been avoiding? What fears, emotions, or memories have been hiding in the background, influencing how I feel about myself and my body?

Losing weight can be straightforward, but shedding emotional and mental barriers may feel more challenging. That's where having a trained coach or guide can make all the difference. Remember, these feelings are rooted in the past—they cannot harm you now. What you're doing is not reliving; it's remembering, and from that place, you can process, release, and heal.

You are not alone on this journey. **You are stronger than you think, and you are ready to move forward.** Let this be the week where you begin to face what has been holding you back, knowing that with every step, you're creating space for the freedom and joy you deserve. You Matter

Key takeaway: Camille realized she wasn't just avoiding food triggers or exercise—she was avoiding the truth. The weight she carried wasn't just physical; it was the weight of unspoken fears, unmet dreams, and unresolved emotions.

Uncovering the Avoidance

Avoidance can be subtle. It hides in our everyday routines, cloaked in distractions, procrastination, and excuses. But deep down, it's often tied to fear—fear of judgment, fear of failure, or fear of the unknown.

Questions to Reflect On:

Before we move into empowerment, we need to acknowledge and explore the areas where avoidance has taken root.

- What things in life have I put off because of my weight?

    o Have you avoided family photos, vacations, or events where you'd feel seen?

- What activities have I been too afraid to try?

    o Is there a dance class, a sport, or even a simple walk in the park you've skipped because you felt self-conscious?

- What relationships have I distanced myself from?

    o Are there people you've avoided because you feel ashamed or not "enough"?

- What dreams have I shelved?

    o Is there a goal, a project, or a passion you've put on hold, telling yourself you'll pursue it "someday"?

Take out your journal and write freely. Let the answers flow without judgment. This is a safe space, to be honest with yourself.

Nike says it best: Just Do ✓ It

The Weight of Avoidance

Avoidance isn't just about the things we don't do—it's about the stories we tell ourselves to justify it. These narratives keep us stuck in a cycle of inaction, feeding our insecurities and reinforcing the belief that we aren't good enough.

These stories often sound like this:

- *"I'm not ready."*

- *"I'll start when I lose 10 pounds."*

- *"People like me don't do that."*

A Moment of Truth:

Camille admitted to avoiding a pottery class she'd dreamed of taking for years. "I kept telling myself I didn't have the time," she said, "but the truth was, I was scared people would judge **me for** how I looked." Once she recognized this, she realized the real weight she carried wasn't on her body—it was in her heart.

Exercise: Diving Into Avoidance

1. List Your Avoidances:

   o Write down all the things you've avoided, big or small, because of your weight or self-doubt.

   o Example: *"I've avoided going to the beach because I hate how I look in a swimsuit."*

2. Identify the Underlying Fear:

    o   For each item, ask yourself: *What am I afraid of?*
        Is it judgment? Failure? Vulnerability?

    o   Example: *"I'm afraid people will stare at me and
        think I don't belong."*

3. Acknowledge the Cost:

    o   What does avoiding these things cost you? Has it
        affected your happiness, relationships, or
        opportunities?

    o   Example: *"I've missed out on precious moments
        with my kids because I didn't want to be in
        photos with them."*

Sitting with Discomfort

Acknowledging avoidance can stir up emotions—guilt, regret,
sadness. That's okay. These feelings are part of the process. By
sitting with them, you begin to release their hold on you.

Take a deep breath and remind yourself: *I am not my past
choices. I have the power to make different ones starting today.*

Preparing for Empowerment

Once you've uncovered what you've been avoiding, the next
step is to reclaim those areas of your life. But first, let's sit with
this question:

*What would my life look like if I stopped avoiding and started
living?*

Write about it. Dream about it. Imagine the joy, freedom, and connection you'd feel if you said yes to the things, you've been saying no to.

Key takeaway: Camille once avoided trying tai chi because she felt self-conscious about her body. But as she released the emotions tied to her weight, she decided to try something new. Today, she finds joy in movement—not because it burns calories but because it makes her feel alive.

Weekly Reflection: What Have You Learned?

Before moving forward, take some time to reflect on what this week has uncovered for you:

- What patterns or fears have surfaced?
- How has avoidance impacted your life?
- What small steps can you take to start reclaiming what you've avoided?

Key takeaway: Like Camille, you might find that the weight you've carried isn't just about food. It could be tied to emotions you've suppressed, relationships you've tolerated, or dreams you've put on hold.

Ask yourself: What am I avoiding? What am I afraid of facing?

Quote to Inspire You

"Avoidance is a great short-term strategy for stress relief, but it's a terrible long-term strategy for happiness." – Dr. Henry Cloud

Fitting comfortably into an airplane or theatre seat, only to travel where you always dreamed of with someone you love. Tackling a big remodeling or landscaping project. How do you want to be living your life in the years ahead? What do you want to be different?

The true first step is taking off your excess weight and keeping it off. This is apt to be the most difficult, exciting, challenging, and rewarding journey of your life.

Your ideal weight is not a step-down or baby-step goal, but rather for you to *Stand Up* for your best weight- your gender, your height, your body frame.

Standing Up for YOU – Because You Matter

Crack the Ego Code

Camille once told me, "I feel like I'm two people. One part of me wants to change, but the other part keeps pulling me back." She was battling her Inner Child, who sought comfort, and her Inner Critic, who shamed her every misstep. Together, we worked to quiet these voices and amplify her Adult Ego—the calm, wise part of her that could lead with love and logic.

Have you ever felt as if you were stuck in an internal battle, fighting yourself over decisions big and small?
"I want that cookie—no, you don't. I want to be healthy—no, I need the cookie now!"

Sound familiar? This tug-of-war happens because we all have three distinct ego states that play a role in our choices:

1. The Inner Child: Sensitive, emotional, and impulsive, this part of us craves immediate pleasure. It doesn't care about long-term consequences; it just wants to feel better *right now.* When you're stressed or sad, the Inner Child often drives you to comfort habits like emotional eating or procrastination.

2. The Adult Ego: Analytical and rational, this is the voice of reason, trying to evaluate situations logically. It wants to guide you toward healthier decisions and long-term goals. However, when it clashes with the Inner Child, it can feel like an exhausting internal argument.

3. The Inner Critic/Parent Ego: This part is judgmental, constantly pointing out your flaws and failures. It believes it's helping you stay on track, but its harsh tone often leads to feelings of guilt, shame, and self-sabotage.

Accepting the Internal Battle

One of the most important steps in healing and releasing weight is acknowledging the inner conflict that often goes unspoken. On the surface, your conscious mind says, *"I want to lose weight. I want to feel confident and healthy."*

But beneath that, your subconscious may be saying…
"If I change, I won't be safe. If I'm seen, I might get hurt."

This tug-of-war isn't weakness—it's protection. Your subconscious is trying to shield you based on past experiences, even if those beliefs no longer serve you. Real transformation begins not by fighting this inner resistance, but by understanding it. When you bring compassion to both parts— the one that wants to move forward and the one that wants to hold back—you create space for healing. This is how change becomes sustainable: not through force, but through awareness, safety, and self-acceptance.

How These Ego States Affect Your Choices

Imagine this scenario: You've had a tough day at work, and all you want is to relax. Your Inner Child whispers, *"You deserve that ice cream; it'll make you feel better."* But as you reach for the freezer, the Adult Ego steps in, saying, *"You've been working so* 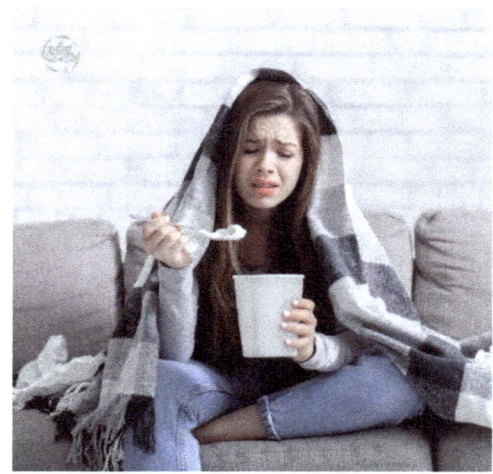 hard to stay healthy—don't do this to yourself!"* Then the Inner Critic chimes in, *"You always give in. Why can't you stick to anything?"*

This battle leaves you drained, frustrated, and often stuck in a cycle of guilt and regret.

But here's the truth: all three ego states have good intentions. The Inner Child wants to soothe you, the Adult Ego wants to protect your goals, and the Inner Critic believes it's motivating you to do better. The key to breaking free lies in awareness and reprogramming these responses.

The Role of Procrastination and Self-Sabotage

Procrastination often stems from the Inner Child's fear of failure or rejection. If you don't try, you can't fail, right? But this avoidance doesn't keep you safe—it keeps you stuck. Similarly, self-sabotage is the Inner Critic's way of protecting you from change. Even maladaptive behaviors have their roots in good intentions: to keep you in your comfort zone where it feels "safe."

Through awareness and tools like hypnosis, you can begin to have a dialogue with these parts of yourself. When you uncover the reasons behind these behaviors, you can shift them in a way that aligns with your goals and values.

Awaken Your Inner Cheerleader

You are more than your Inner Critic's harsh words. You have strengths, accomplishments, and resilience waiting to be recognized. Replacing your Inner Critic with an internal cheerleader doesn't happen overnight, but it starts with small steps. Begin by speaking to yourself with kindness:

- Instead of: *"I can't believe I messed up again."*

    o   Try: *"I'm learning and growing every day."*

- Instead of: *"I'll never lose this weight."*

    o   Try: *"I'm making choices that support my health and happiness."*

Your ego states are not your enemies—they're parts of you that need understanding, compassion, and guidance. As you work to reprogram these patterns, you'll find it easier to make choices that honor your goals and values.

Note on Transformation

When you change how you speak to yourself, you change the way you show up in the world. Hypnosis and self-awareness allow you to bypass old programming and create new pathways that support your evolution.
Remember, shedding weight isn't just about your body—it's about freeing yourself to live authentically in every part of your life.

"For me, shedding the weight means freeing yourself to tell the truth and be the truth in every spectrum of your life." ~ Oprah

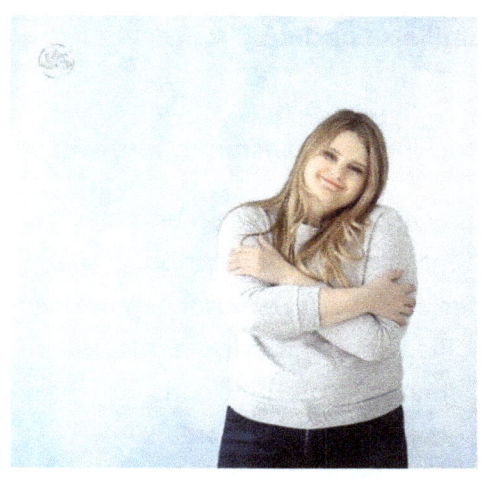

WEEK SEVEN - Focus: Embracing Self-Compassion

This week is all about embracing—embracing who you are, where you've been, and where you're going. Now that you've evoked past patterns and limiting beliefs, it's time to offer yourself the kindness and compassion you deserve.

Emotional Issue of Being Overweight

In Week 6, you began exploring what you've been avoiding and how facing those emotions can lead to profound transformation. Now, let's focus on resilience—the ability to bounce back, adapt, and grow stronger in the face of challenges.

What Is Resilience?

Resilience is not about avoiding hardships; it's about navigating through them with grace and determination. It's the inner strength that allows you to persevere, even when the road feels uncertain. Camille, whom you met in Week 4, is a shining example of resilience. At 70, she faced decades of self-doubt and toxic relationships. Through her journey, she not only transformed her body but also rebuilt her life.

119

The Power of Resilience: Camille's Continued Journey

This week, we'll explore how to cultivate your resilience and use it as a tool to support your ongoing transformation.

Camille didn't wake up one day and suddenly feel empowered. Her journey required consistent effort, self-reflection, and a willingness to step outside her comfort zone. After separating from her toxic marriage, Camille experienced moments of fear and doubt. But she chose to channel those emotions into activities that nurtured her soul—tai chi, art classes, and swimming. Each step she took reinforced her resilience and deepened her belief in her ability to thrive.

Like Camille, you have the power to build resilience. It starts with small, intentional actions that reaffirm your inner strength and capacity for change.

Building Resilience Through Awareness

To cultivate resilience, you must first become aware of how you respond to challenges. Do you avoid them? Do you face them head-on? Do you criticize yourself when things don't go as planned?

Exercise: Recognizing Your Resilience Patterns

Take a moment to reflect on the following questions:

1. **When faced with a challenge, how do I typically respond?**

   - Example: Do you freeze, overthink, or take immediate action?

2. **What's one challenge I've overcome in the past, and how did I navigate it?**

   - Example: Think about a time you solved a problem, big or small. What strengths did you use?

3. **What negative self-talk arises during difficult moments, and how can I reframe it?**

   - Example: Replace "I can't handle this" with "I've faced hard things before, and I'll get through this too."

Write your answers in your journal. Celebrate your past successes and acknowledge the resilience you've already shown.

Resilience and the Subconscious Mind

Your subconscious mind plays a significant role in how you perceive challenges. If you've internalized beliefs like "I'm not strong enough" or "I always fail," those thoughts will influence your actions. But just as you've learned to reprogram other patterns, you can teach your subconscious to embrace resilience.

Affirmation Exercise: Rewiring for Resilience

Each day this week, practice these affirmations:

- "I am stronger than I realize."

- "Every challenge I face helps me grow."

- "I have the tools to navigate any situation."

Say these affirmations out loud in front of a mirror, with conviction. Repeat them throughout the day, especially when facing a difficult moment. Over time, these positive statements will become part of your subconscious programming.

Action Steps: Strengthening Your Resilience

1. **Set a Micro-Goal:** Choose one small action that challenges you this week. It could be trying a new workout, saying no to a tempting but unhealthy food choice, or having an honest conversation you've been avoiding.

2. **Create a Resilience Ritual:** Develop a daily practice that grounds you. This might include deep breathing, journaling, or a short walk to clear your mind.

3. **Connect With Your Support System:** Share your journey with a trusted friend, coach, or group. Knowing you're not alone can bolster your confidence and motivation.

4. **Celebrate Small Wins:** At the end of each day, write down one thing you did well. It could be as simple as drinking more water, resisting a negative thought, or showing up for yourself.

Reflection: The Lessons of Resilience

As you move through Week 7, remember that resilience isn't about perfection. It's about showing up, even when it feels hard, and trusting that each small step brings you closer to the life you deserve.

Take a moment to reflect on what resilience means to you. Write it down. Then, consider how embracing resilience can support your journey of transformation.

Quote to Inspire

"Do not judge me by my success, judge me by how many times I fell down and got back up again." ~ Nelson Mandela

Looking Ahead

Next week, we'll focus on deepening your connection with your inner wisdom and intuition. Together, we'll explore how to trust yourself fully and use that trust to guide your decisions. For now, continue building your resilience and know that every step you take matters.

With so many people making demands on you, it may feel impossible to take time for yourself. Perhaps you've been told 'don't be selfish,' 'place your own needs last,' and 'give until it hurts' or 'isn't that a bit selfish of you'?

If you have created a situation in which there seems to be no time for yourself, recognize that no one forced you, but you created or agreed to it. You took it upon yourself to repeat or honor their words.

The job or family members did not come along and place those demands upon you. You allowed it to happen. Or you asked for it.

Complete this sentence - I feel worthy when

_____

Recognizing Your Patterns and Making New Choices

Congratulations on making it to this pivotal part of your journey. By now, you've uncovered some truths about yourself—patterns, emotions, and beliefs that have shaped your relationship with your body. This week, let's talk about a deeper truth: **Why is it so hard to put yourself first?**

Think about the messages you've heard throughout your life:

- "Don't be selfish."

- "Place your own needs last."

- "Give until it hurts."

- "Isn't that a bit selfish of you?"

These words often echo in our minds long after they've been spoken, shaping the choices we make and the roles we take on. Over time, you may have found yourself agreeing to demands, saying "yes" when you meant "no," or believing that your worth comes from how much you give to others. But here's the truth: **No one forced you into this.** Somewhere along the way, you chose to honor those words, perhaps out of love, fear, or a desire for approval.

What Makes You Feel Worthy?

Take a moment to complete this sentence:
I feel worthy when _____.

Did you answer with something like, "When I'm helping others" or "When I'm useful"? If so, you're not alone. Many of us equate our worth with what we can do for others. We strive for love and acceptance, believing that if we just give enough, we'll be enough. This belief is rooted in a universal fear: the fear of losing love or approval. To truly thrive, you must begin to recognize your inherent worth, independent of what you do for others.

Facing the Inner Dialogue

Let's pause and examine the voices within you. We all have three ego states:

1. **The Inner Child:** Sensitive, emotional, and reactive. It craves comfort and reassurance.

2. **The Inner Critic/Parent Ego:** Judgmental and critical. It enforces rules and expectations.

3. **The Adult Ego:** Rational, balanced, and compassionate. It helps us navigate life with clarity.

Ask yourself:

- When you make choices, who is in charge?

- Is it the Inner Self (child) throwing a tantrum, seeking instant gratification?

- Is it the Inner Critic, scolding you for not being good enough?

- Or is it the Adult Ego, making decisions from a place of self-love and awareness?

Becoming aware of these voices is the first step toward reclaiming your power. When you recognize who's speaking, you can consciously choose to respond differently.

Empowering Through Self-Awareness

There is something deeply powerful about a woman who begins to truly understand herself. As you recognize the patterns that have shaped your behavior, emotional eating, self-sabotage, or negative self-talk, you're no longer blaming yourself; you're awakening. This isn't about guilt or shame—it's about taking gentle responsibility. You're choosing to be honest, vulnerable, and compassionate with yourself, knowing that true growth comes from awareness, not judgment.

By listening to your mind, honoring your emotions, and respecting your body, you're creating a new way of being—one rooted in kindness, strength, and personal truth. This is the path to lasting transformation: not perfection, but presence. Not control, just connection!

Embracing Menopause – Honoring Your Body Through the Change

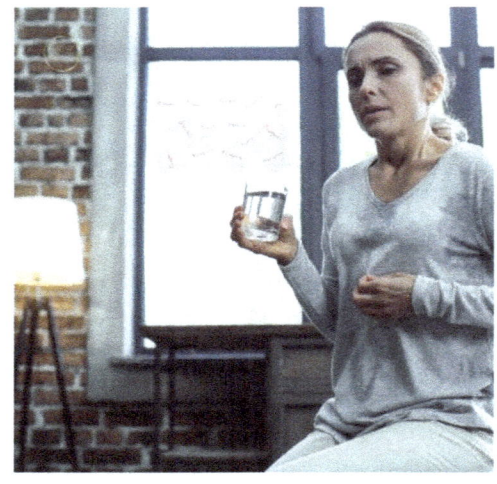

Menopause is a profound transition, a natural phase in every woman's life that often feels like an emotional, mental, and physical rollercoaster. For many, it's a time of grief, self-reflection, and even confusion.

Society has often shrouded menopause in silence, portraying it as the end of youth, desirability, and vitality. But this chapter is here to tell you otherwise. Menopause isn't the end—it's an awakening, a new chapter that offers opportunities to redefine how you see yourself and your body.

The Emotional Journey

Menopause often triggers feelings of loss. The inability to bear children may feel like losing a part of your identity as a woman. Add to this the hormonal shifts that affect mood, and it's no wonder that many women feel emotionally turbulent during this time. You might experience mood swings, irritability, sadness, or even anger. These emotions are valid and worth honoring, but they do not define you.

It's also common to struggle with self-worth during menopause. Changes in your body—whether it's bloating, weight gain, or sagging skin—can lead to feelings of unattractiveness. Sexual desire may wane, leaving you questioning your desirability and femininity. But let me remind you: you are no less a woman than you were before. This is a time to nurture yourself and connect with the essence of who you are beyond societal definitions.

The Physical Changes

Menopause brings with it a slew of physical changes that can feel overwhelming. Hot flashes, night sweats, fatigue, and bloating may leave you feeling uncomfortable in your skin. The decline in estrogen levels affects everything from your skin's elasticity to bone health. Sexual desire may fluctuate, leaving you feeling disconnected from your body or your partner.

These physical changes are not a betrayal by your body; they are simply transitions. Your body, after decades of serving you, is asking for a different kind of care and attention.

How Hypnosis Can Help

Hypnosis is a powerful tool for navigating menopause. It helps address emotional struggles by rewiring negative thought patterns and promoting feelings of acceptance and empowerment. Hypnosis can also provide relief from physical symptoms, such as reducing the intensity and frequency of hot flashes or managing sleep disturbances.

Through guided visualization, hypnosis can help you reconnect with your body, replacing frustration with gratitude and discomfort with ease. Hypnosis isn't about ignoring the symptoms—it's about transforming how you experience them.

Holistic Approaches for Menopause

In addition to hypnosis, there are other holistic approaches to support your journey:

1. Nutrition: Eat a balanced diet rich in phytoestrogens (like soy and flaxseed) to help balance hormones naturally.

2. Movement: Gentle exercises like yoga, tai chi, or walking can reduce stress, improve bone health, and enhance mood.

3. Naturopathy: Consider herbal remedies such as black cohosh, red clover, or evening primrose oil under the guidance of a healthcare provider.

4. Mindfulness and Meditation: Deep breathing, mindfulness, and meditation can reduce stress and emotional turbulence.

5. Hydration: Drink plenty of water to counteract bloating and improve skin health.

6. Community: Join a support group or connect with other women going through similar experiences. Knowing you're not alone can be incredibly comforting.

Honoring Your Body

Menopause isn't something to battle; it's something to honor. It's a signal from your body that it's time to turn inward, to focus on nurturing and sustaining yourself. Your body has carried you through decades of life—it deserves care, love, and respect during this transition.

Celebrate the wisdom that comes with age. Celebrate the freedom of no longer worrying about periods or contraception. Celebrate the ability to prioritize your needs and desires in a way that might not have been possible before.

Repeat affirmations that foster acceptance and empowerment:

- "I honor my body's wisdom as it evolves."
- "I release the need for external validation and embrace inner peace."

Coping Strategies for Emotional Struggles

1. Acknowledge Your Feelings: It's okay to feel sad, frustrated, or even angry. Allow yourself to process these emotions without judgment.

2. Seek Support: Talk to a therapist, hypnotherapist, or trusted friend who can help you navigate your feelings.

3. Self-Care Rituals: Pamper yourself with massages, warm baths, or journaling to cultivate a sense of peace.

4. Sharing your journey with others—it's both healing and empowering.

You Are Evolving

Menopause marks the end of one chapter but the beginning of another. It's an opportunity to evolve into a version of yourself that is freer, wiser, and more attuned to your needs. You are not defined by the ability to bear children, your youthful appearance, or societal expectations. You are defined by your resilience, your kindness, your wisdom, and your capacity to grow.

Embrace this time with the grace and strength that only a woman like you can possess. Menopause isn't an ending—it's your evolution.

Healing and Moving Forward

Healing begins with honesty. As Oprah once said:

"Unless you fix the trauma that has caused people to be the way they are...you are working on the wrong thing."

You cannot fix a weight issue without addressing the underlying emotional wounds and beliefs. This means acknowledging the fears, hurts, and unspoken truths you've carried for so long. Remember, these emotions are part of your past—they cannot harm you now. They are simply memories, and you are stronger than them.

Ask yourself:

- What am I afraid of letting go of?

- What beliefs or patterns am I clinging to, even though they no longer serve me?

A New Way Forward

Change isn't about quick fixes. It's about making choices from a place of self-awareness and self-respect. This means shifting from **reaction** to **intention**:

- Instead of dieting to "fix" yourself, nurture your body because you love it.

- Instead of exercising out of guilt, move your body to celebrate what it can do.

- Instead of hiding behind excuses, step into your power and take responsibility for your happiness.

Your body reflects your life—physical, emotional, intellectual, and spiritual. When one aspect is out of balance, it affects the whole. True transformation happens when you honor all parts of yourself and commit to living in alignment with your values and desires.

A Gentle Reminder

Imagine wearing shoes that are too tight. At first, you tolerate the discomfort, convincing yourself that it's not so bad. But over time, the pain worsens, affecting your posture, your balance, and your overall well-being. The only way to heal is to take off the shoes and allow your feet to breathe.

Your weight and the emotions tied to it are like those tight shoes. The pain won't go away until you address the root cause. But when you do, you'll discover a freedom and lightness you never thought possible.

Reflection Questions

Take some time to journal your thoughts:

1. What emotions have I been avoiding?

2. How have I been seeking validation or worth from others?

3. What would it look like to prioritize my needs without guilt or fear?

4. How can I honor all four aspects of myself—physical, emotional, intellectual, and spiritual?

Quote of the Week:

"Forgiveness is the fragrance that the violet sheds on the heel that has crushed it." – Mark Twain

Final Thoughts

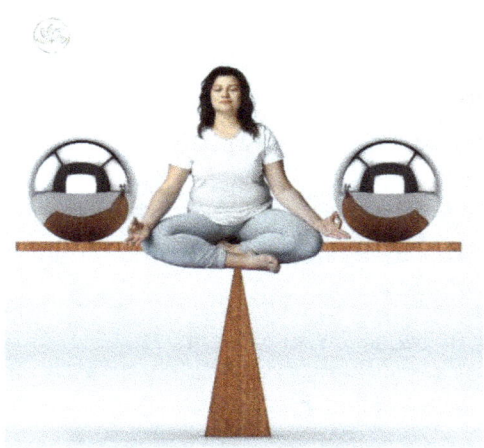

Happiness is a balancing act—a dance between holding on and letting go. As you move forward, remember that every small step you take toward self-love and self-awareness is a victory. You are not alone on this journey. I am here to guide and support you because you matter.

And always keep in mind: **"You are not your body—but your body is yours."**

Did you complete the sentence with some version of... When I help others? When doing good for others... When am I useful?

We all strive for love and acceptance. The foundation of every person who gives and gives and gives is the fundamental belief that if they just do enough and do it well enough, then they will be loved. The deep-seated fear of loss of love or loss of approval is almost universal.

So much of what we do is a reaction to past patterns and conditioning. To change conditioning, think of the 3 Egos. Is your reaction being a loving adult, or is the inner child having a tantrum, or is your inner critic being loud and critical?

A change as fundamental as your body image, especially if you are talking about a significant amount of weight, is not going to be possible in an atmosphere where the unspoken contract is one of keeping things hidden inside and the same.

Once you begin to recognize how you react, it becomes easier to work on loving yourself. This may happen over time, and it may also be difficult until you get to recognize it faster, but it is always worth loving you. Because… You Matter.

Resilience Through Self-Forgiveness: A Client's Story

Self-forgiveness can be one of the most challenging yet liberating steps in your journey. It often feels easier to forgive others for their shortcomings than to extend the same compassion to ourselves. But forgiveness—true, deep forgiveness—starts within.

Let me tell you about Katherine. She spent most of her married life as the sole provider for her family. Her husband was angry and controlling, struggling with alcoholism, while Katherine worked tirelessly to support their three children and care for her ailing brother and parents. For years, she dismissed her own needs, carrying the burdens of her family on her shoulders.

When Katherine came to me, she was in a state of physical and emotional depletion. Her husband was in the hospital, nearing the end of his life, and Katherine was experiencing debilitating panic attacks. Over the last decade, she had gained more than

47 pounds, a result of stress, emotional eating, and the weight of unprocessed emotions.

The Journey to Forgiveness

Not so easy. Self-forgiveness can be harder than forgiving others.

Through our sessions, Katherine began to unravel the layers of pain and resentment she had carried since childhood. She shared memories of hiding in a closet with her brother, clutching a box of cookies while their mother endured domestic violence in the next room. That box of cookies became their only source of comfort, setting the stage for Katherine's later relationship with food.

When we began working together, Katherine was quick to forgive her husband for his troubled past but resisted forgiving herself. She blamed herself for her weight gain, for "letting things happen," and for not feeling worthy of love or happiness.

Through hypnosis and guided exploration, Katherine began to see the blueprint of her life—the patterns and beliefs that had shaped her decisions. She realized her weight was not just physical; it was a manifestation of the burdens she had carried for years. Slowly, she started to forgive herself—not for gaining weight, but for the unrealistic expectations she had placed on herself and for the ways she had dismissed her own needs.

The Transformation

By the end of our nine-week sessions, Katherine had dropped 19 pounds—not just from her body but from her spirit. She found clarity, letting go of the guilt and resentment that had weighed her down for decades. More importantly, she reclaimed her sense of worth and began prioritizing herself.

Your Turn: Reflect on Forgiveness

As you read Katherine's story, ask yourself:

- Is there something you've been holding onto that you haven't forgiven yourself for?

- How has that affected your relationship with yourself and your body?

Take a moment to journal your thoughts. Write about a time when you felt you "failed" yourself. Then, write a letter of forgiveness to yourself. Be kind. Be honest. Remember, forgiveness isn't about erasing the past—it's about freeing yourself to move forward.

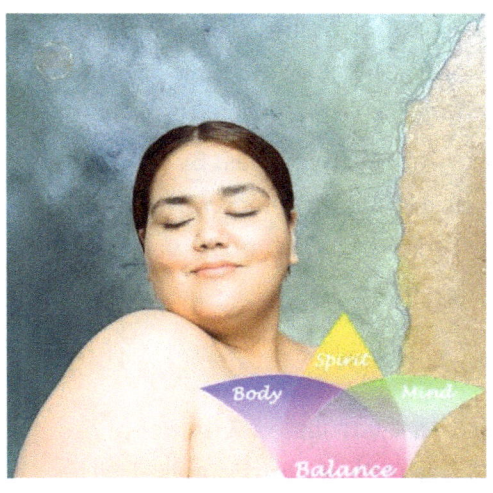

WEEK EIGHT - Shake hands with your subconscious mind– The Week of Harmony

Congratulations on reaching Week 8! This is the week of harmony—a time to deepen your connection with your subconscious mind and align it with your conscious desires. By now, you've evoked deep awareness, embraced the truths about yourself, and begun evolving into the empowered individual you are meant to be. This week, we focus on unifying the parts of yourself that may have felt at odds for years.

Your subconscious mind is not a separate entity—it's a powerful partner in your transformation. When you learn to work with it, rather than against it, the results can be life-changing.

What Does It Mean to Shake Hands with Your Subconscious Mind?

Imagine your subconscious mind as a dear friend—one who holds your deepest memories, emotions, and habits. This friend wants to protect you and help you survive, but sometimes they misinterpret what you truly need. For example, your subconscious might associate eating cookies with comfort because, at one point, that's what helped you cope. This week, you'll learn how to harmonize with your subconscious, transforming old patterns into supportive ones. By shaking hands with your subconscious mind, you're acknowledging its role in your life and inviting it to work with you toward your goals.

Camille's Subconscious Breakthrough

Camille, whom you met in Week 4, struggled with deeply ingrained patterns rooted in decades of emotional pain. Her subconscious mind had linked food to safety, companionship, and relief. Together, we worked to help her "introduce herself" to her subconscious. Through guided visualization, she acknowledged the ways her subconscious had been trying to help her and lovingly reprogrammed those patterns.

By working with her subconscious rather than battling it, Camille began to make choices that supported her well-being. Her transformation wasn't just physical; it was emotional and spiritual. Camille discovered that harmony within herself was the key to lasting change.

The Subconscious Mind: A Powerful Partner

Your subconscious mind operates like a GPS. If it's programmed with outdated or faulty coordinates, you'll keep arriving at destinations you don't want. To recalibrate, you need to communicate clearly and consistently with your subconscious.

Here's the good news: Your subconscious mind does not judge. It accepts whatever you feed it as truth, whether positive or negative. The key is to nourish it with empowering thoughts, imagery, and emotions.

Exercise: Meet Your Subconscious

1. **Find a Quiet Space:** Sit comfortably, close your eyes, and take three deep breaths. Let your body relax completely.

2. **Visualize Your Subconscious Mind:** Imagine your subconscious as a wise guide or a trusted friend. What do they look like? How do they greet you?

3. **Start a Conversation:** Silently or out loud, thank your subconscious for always protecting you and keeping you safe. Then, share your current goals. For example, "I am grateful for your support as I create a healthier, lighter version of myself."

4. **Listen:** Pause and notice any thoughts, feelings, or images that arise. This is your subconscious mind's way of communicating with you.

Repeat this exercise daily. Over time, you'll strengthen your bond and feel more aligned with your inner self.

Action Steps for Harmonizing with Your Subconscious

1. **Rewrite Your Inner Narrative:** Choose one limiting belief you've held about yourself and replace it with a positive affirmation. For example, change "I'll never lose this weight" to "My body is becoming healthier every day."

2. **Visualize Success:** Spend 5 minutes each day imagining your ideal self. See yourself walking confidently, feeling light, and radiating joy. The clearer the image, the more powerfully your subconscious will respond.

3. **Practice Gratitude:** Each night, write down three things your body has done for you that day. Gratitude reinforces a loving partnership with your subconscious mind.

4. **Create a Trigger for Harmony:** Choose a small, symbolic gesture—like placing your hand on your heart or tapping your wrist—that reminds you to connect with your subconscious. Use this gesture whenever you need encouragement or focus.

Embracing Harmony

This week, allow yourself to let go of internal conflict. Embrace the harmony that comes from aligning your conscious and subconscious minds. When these two parts of yourself work together, the results are profound and lasting.

Looking Ahead

Next week, we'll complete this transformative journey by focusing on evolving fully into the person you've been working so hard to become. For now, take time to honor the connection you're building with your subconscious mind. Harmony is within reach—you just need to reach out and grasp it.

Why Do We Eat the Way We Do?

In Week Eight, you explored how your subconscious mind influences your eating habits and emotional responses to food. This section dives deeper into the root causes behind these patterns, helping you recognize and reprogram them.

1. You Eat to Reward or Entertain Yourself

From infancy, we associate food with comfort and reward. A cookie for good behavior, a celebratory dinner for a special occasion, or ice cream after a tough day—these patterns become deeply ingrained in our subconscious. Over time, food becomes a substitute for emotional fulfillment.

Reframe: Recognize moments when you use food as a reward. Can you replace it with non-food-related rewards? For example, a relaxing bath, a favorite song, or a quiet walk.

2. You Eat to Lessen the Pain

When emotional or physical discomfort arises, food often feels like a quick fix. Think of a child given a treat to distract from teething pain or an adult seeking solace in ice cream after a rough day. However, this comfort is fleeting, and the underlying hurt remains.

3. You Eat to Command Attention

For some, food serves as a means to be noticed or to take up space in the world. A larger body might feel like a protective shield or a way to assert significance.

Reframe: Reflect on your inner voice. Are you equating size with importance? How can you command attention in other ways, such as through self-expression or confidence?

4. You Eat When You Need Love

This may be the hardest truth to confront. When love feels inaccessible, food often becomes the substitute. It provides a sense of self-soothing but can also perpetuate cycles of loneliness and self-loathing.

Reframe: Begin practicing self-love. Use affirmations like, "I am worthy of love just as I am," and explore ways to nurture yourself outside of food.

5. You Eat Because of Fear

Fear of being seen, judged, or vulnerable can lead to overeating. By burying your true self beneath layers of weight, you may feel protected but also trapped.

Reframe: Ask yourself, "What am I afraid of facing?" Write it down. Acknowledge the fear and then visualize yourself letting it go.

Listen to Your Body Talk

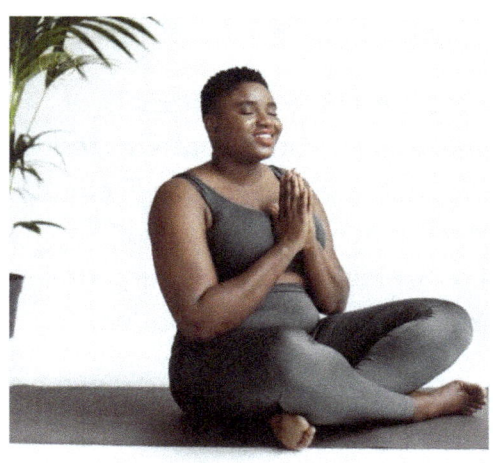

Your body is always communicating with you—when you feel hot or cold, pleasure or pain, it's your body speaking. But in the hustle of life— working, socializing, eating, dancing, or simply going about your day—it's easy to take your body for granted. Often, we only notice its signals when they become undeniable, like illness, fatigue, or discomfort.

However, dissociation from your body robs you of the joy of being present in it. It's like looking at yourself in a mirror and feeling a disconnect, as though the reflection is you, yet somehow distant. This disconnect can develop for many reasons—trauma, stress, or simply years of ignoring your body's subtle messages.

For some, this dissociation manifests as stuffing emotions into their body. Perhaps you've ignored or denied the pain and hurt you've felt, thinking it would go away on its own. Eventually, those unaddressed emotions will surface, often in ways that feel familiar but are undesirable—such as overeating, chronic fatigue, or even physical pain.

The Subconscious and the 3 Egos

Remember the concept of the 3 Egos? The subconscious, or inner child, is where emotional triggers and old patterns reside. When the inner child perceives a threat—real or imagined—it commands a "run" response, prompting you to flee both physically and psychologically. For many, this flight response involves reaching for comfort foods or numbing emotions.

Meanwhile, the parent ego steps in to protect you, but it often reinforces maladaptive behaviors like overeating, smoking, or self-loathing. These behaviors may have served a purpose once—perhaps shielding you from deeper pain—but they no longer serve the empowered, authentic version of you that you are becoming.

By defending past trauma through these behaviors, you unintentionally create new layers of trauma. Over time, this cycle perpetuates feelings of guilt, shame, and disconnection.

Reconnecting With Your Body

Are you ready to take back control of your life? To care for yourself deeply and respect the incredible being that you are? Here's how you can start:

- Let go of old habits that block your true feelings. Recognize them for what they are—coping mechanisms—and release their hold on you.

- Identify unhealthy habits that have cushioned you but no longer serve your highest good. This might include overeating, smoking, oversleeping, or other behaviors that deny your authentic self.

- Create a safe space where you can process emotions. This might be a quiet room, a favorite nature spot, or a trusted friend's home.

Allow Yourself to Feel

As you let go of these habits, suppressed emotions may begin to surface—anger, hurt, or sadness. Allow yourself to feel them. Cry if you need to. Laugh. Scream. Let the knots of tension unravel. This process may be difficult at first, but it's also liberating. Listening to your body talk is an act of self-trust and acceptance.

The key is to remember: You have a choice, and you deserve better. Each time you choose to honor your body's needs; you take a step toward greater harmony and self-love.

Tools to Reconnect

The 'Stand Up to Slim Down' Program is designed to help you rebuild this connection. By combining hypnosis, conscious programming, and practical tools, it empowers you to change your habits and mindset effortlessly, painlessly, and permanently.

Through this program, you'll learn to:

- Recognize and honor your body's signals.

- Replace outdated patterns with empowering choices.

- Develop a deeper connection with yourself—physically, emotionally, and mentally.

Consider exploring one of our live workshops, where we dive even deeper into these concepts. You'll learn how to build a lifelong partnership with your body, guided by expert tools and support.

Rewriting Your Subconscious Story

Your body is not separate from your mind, but a reflection of it. When you think, "I hate my body," your subconscious takes that as a directive. Let's rewrite that narrative:

- Replace "I hate my body" with "I appreciate my body for all it does for me."

- Replace "I'll never lose this weight" with "I am becoming healthier every day."

Reflection Questions:

- What emotions are you stuffing with food?

- What habits are protecting you but no longer serve your higher self?

- How can you create new rituals that honor your emotional and physical needs?

Quote of the Week:

"The body achieves what the mind believes." ~ Napoleon Hill

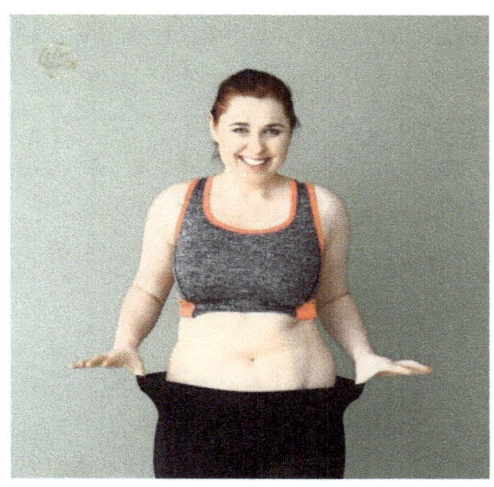

WEEK NINE - Evolving into Your Best Self

Congratulations!

You've made it to Week 9— the number for completion and transformation. This is your moment to celebrate how far you've come. You've evoked what was and embraced what is, and now it's time to evolve into what will be.

Think about the courage, effort, and commitment you've shown over these past weeks. This journey hasn't been about perfection but about progress, self-discovery, and creating a foundation for lasting change.

You are here because you matter, and this is your time to shine.

Listen to Your Body Talk: Connecting to Your Inner Wisdom

Your body has been your silent companion, carrying the weight of your experiences, emotions, and stories. It whispers to you in sensations—warmth, chills, tension, or lightness—but often, in the hustle and bustle of life, these whispers are drowned out. This week, we focus on reconnecting with your body, listening to its messages, and nurturing the partnership between your mind and body.

149

Dissociation from your body can rob you of the joy of truly inhabiting yourself. It's as if you are seeing yourself in a mirror but standing too far away to feel connected. Perhaps you've been stuffing emotions into your body, pretending the pain or hurt wasn't there. But your body doesn't forget—it carries the stories you've tried to bury, waiting patiently for you to listen.

Understanding Emotional Eating Patterns

1. **Eating as a Reward or Entertainment:** From childhood, food is often tied to emotions. We celebrate achievements with treats or soothe teething pain with biscuits. As adults, food remains a comfort during celebrations and a balm during difficult times. But when eating becomes an automatic response to every emotion, it stops serving us.

2. **Eating to Escape or Numb Pain:** Have you ever reached for ice cream after heartbreak or chips after a long, stressful day? These patterns, ingrained since childhood, feel comforting now but don't resolve the underlying hurt.

3. **Eating for Attention:** Sometimes, overeating or holding onto weight can be a subconscious way of demanding attention or creating a sense of importance. It becomes a way to fill a void when self-worth feels diminished.

4. **Eating as a Substitute for Love:** Food can become a stand-in for affection. When we're starved for love, we may turn to the comfort of a full plate, trying to fill an emotional emptiness.

5. **Eating Out of Fear:** Fear of being seen, judged, or desired can lead some to overeat as a protective mechanism, hiding their true selves beneath layers of weight.

Releasing Old Habits and Emotions

To reconnect with your body, you must let go of the habits that no longer serve you. These habits—overeating, oversleeping, procrastinating—may have protected you in the past, but now they weigh you down.

- **Acknowledge Your Feelings:** It's okay to feel hurt, angry, or overwhelmed. Allow these feelings to surface without judgment.

- **Create a Safe Space:** Find a quiet spot where you can process your emotions, whether it's your room, a garden, or even a yoga mat.

- **Release Through Movement:** Dance, walk, or stretch. Let your body express what words cannot.

Mindful Exercises to Reconnect

Cleansing with Water: A Ritual of Renewal

Water is one of the purest elements in nature, carrying both physical and symbolic power.

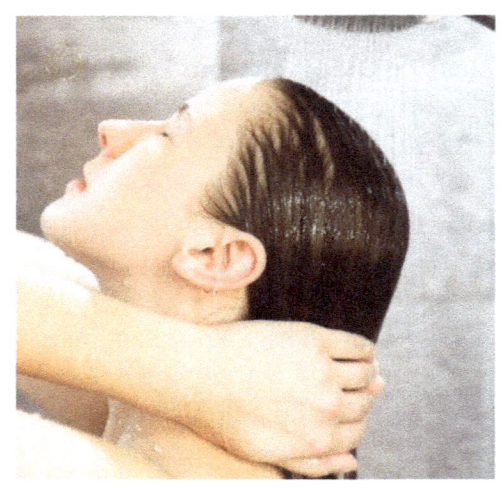

As you step into a warm shower, you're not just washing your body; you're engaging in a timeless ritual of cleansing and renewal.

Think about it—water has been there in every stage of your life. As a child, you were bathed with care, held, and pampered. Those moments weren't just about cleanliness; they were about love, nurturing, and the sense of being cherished.

Now, as you stand under the flowing water, you have the power to create that same sense of care for yourself. This is your time to let go—to cleanse not only your skin but also your mind and spirit. Picture the water as it cascades over you. Each drop is a messenger, gently washing away the pain, hurt, and old memories you no longer need to carry. Imagine the worries that weigh on your heart, the stress of the day swirling down the drain.

Speak to yourself with kindness. Repeat affirmations to deepen this release:

- "I let go of all that no longer serves me and welcome renewal and clarity."

- "I let the flowing water clear away my worries and pain."

- "I allow the water to wash away all that no longer serves me."

- "I am restored and balanced, ready for a fresh start."

Let the water soothe you, just as it did when you were a child, and let yourself feel pampered, nurtured, and held by its warmth. If tears come, let them flow—they're part of the release. If a song bubbles up, sing it loud and free. This is your moment to reset, to shed what's heavy, and to step out feeling lighter, clearer, and more balanced.

Water is life's purest element, and with it, you can cleanse not just your body but the energy that surrounds and fills you. Today, as you shower, give yourself this gift of renewal. **You deserve it.**

Discover Your Inner Switch

Your body holds the power to relax and release:

- **The Green Switch:** Imagine a green switch in your mind. When you turn it off, your muscles release tension. Practice turning it on and off, noticing how your body responds.

- **The Blue Switch:** This switch slows your thoughts, quieting the noise in your mind. Visualize floating clouds carrying your worries away as you turn this switch off.

Visualization: Seeing Your Best Self

Visualization is a powerful tool to align your subconscious mind with your goals. Here's how to create a vivid image of your transformed self:

1. **Close Your Eyes and Picture It:** See yourself at your ideal weight. What are you wearing? How do you feel? Notice the confidence in your posture and the lightness in your movements.

2. **Engage All Your Senses:** Hear the sound of your laughter, feel the texture of your clothes, and notice the joy radiating from within.

3. **Own the Feeling:** Repeat affirmations like, *"I am becoming my best self every day. I am strong, capable, and worthy."*

Your Words Shape Your Reality

Remember, we talked about words. The words you use have immense power over your body and mind. Replace phrases like "I don't know" with *"I'm allowing myself to uncover the answers."* Your subconscious is always listening—choose words that uplift and empower you.

- Instead of *"I'm fat,"* say, *"I am on a health journey."*

- Instead of *"I can't do this,"* say, *"I'm learning and growing every day."*

Action Steps for This Week

1. **Track Your Patterns:** Keep a journal of when and why you eat. Are you truly hungry, or are you responding to an emotion?

2. **Drink Water Mindfully:** Each time you drink, imagine it cleansing your body and mind, washing away negativity.

3. **Practice the Visualization Exercise Daily:** Reinforce your new image of yourself.

4. **Affirmations:** Use empowering phrases to reprogram your mind and nurture your confidence.

Quote of the Week

"You can't do anything that you can't picture yourself doing." – Anonymous

Workshops for Deeper Connection

If this week's exercises resonated with you, consider joining one of our *Listen to Your Body Talk* workshops. These sessions dive deeper into reconnecting with your body, releasing emotional weight, and cultivating a lifelong partnership with yourself.

You're not just shedding pounds—you're shedding old stories, habits, and limitations. You are evolving into your best self, one mindful choice at a time.

Reflection: Acknowledge the Journey

Let's take a moment to reflect on the milestones you've achieved:

- You've evoked old patterns and beliefs that were holding you back.

- You've embraced your present reality with compassion and curiosity.

- You've taken steps to rewrite your story, shedding physical and emotional weight.

Transformation isn't just about what's on the outside. It's about becoming aligned—body, mind, and spirit. Each choice you've made has been a step toward the life you deserve.

You Matter!

Stepping Into Your New Chapter

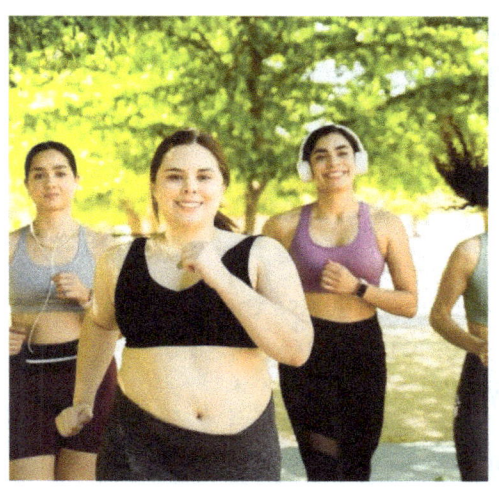

The process of evolving isn't about "fixing" yourself; it's about uncovering the strength, resilience, and beauty that have always been within you. Like a butterfly emerging from its chrysalis, you've done the inner work, and now it's time to soar. But evolution doesn't end here—it's a continuous journey. As you move forward, consider this a time to solidify your new habits, embrace new possibilities, and continue honoring your true self.

Exercise: Visualizing Your Evolved Self

1. **Find a Quiet Space:** Sit comfortably, close your eyes, and take a few deep breaths. Allow yourself to relax and center your thoughts.

2. **Picture Your Future Self:** Imagine yourself six months or a year from now. What does your life look like? How do you feel in your body? What are you doing? Who are you surrounded by?

3. **Engage Your Senses:** What do you see, hear, and feel in this future version of yourself? Notice the joy, confidence, and ease in your evolved self.

4. **Write It Down:** Open your journal and describe this vision in detail. Use affirming language such as "I am," "I feel," and "I have."

Affirmation for the Week

"I am proud of the work I've done. I release the past, embrace the present, and step confidently into my future. I am evolving into the best version of myself."

Remember, you're not alone. If you ever feel the need for guidance or encouragement, I'm here for you!

Action Steps for Sustaining Your Evolution

1. **Celebrate Your Wins:** Acknowledge and reward yourself for your progress. Whether it's a heartfelt note of gratitude to yourself or treating yourself to a new outfit that reflects your transformation, make it meaningful.

2. **Practice Daily Gratitude:** Each morning or evening, write down three things you're grateful for. Gratitude keeps you grounded and focused on the positive.

3. **Embrace Lifelong Learning:** Keep growing by reading, attending workshops, or exploring new interests. **Share Your Story:** Your journey can inspire others. Whether you write about it, talk about it, or simply share it with those close to you, let your transformation shine.

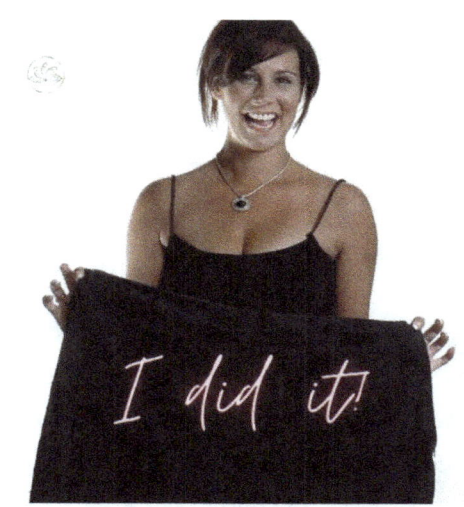

Congratulations!

You Did It!

This is your time to celebrate not just the completion of a program but the beginning of a new chapter in your life.

You've stood up, let go, and slimmed down—not just in body but in spirit. You've proven to yourself that change is possible, and you are deserving of the love, joy, and freedom that come with it.

Here's to your continued evolution—because **You Matter!**

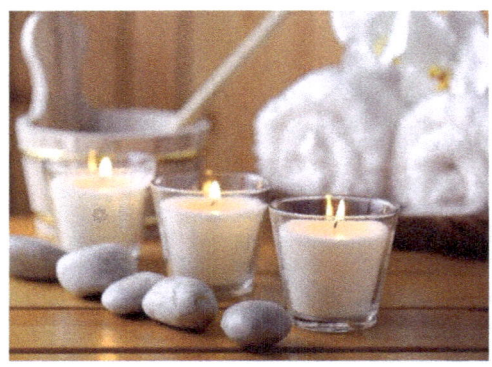

Liza's '33 Days' New Habit-Forming Theory:

You may have heard the phrase "It takes 21 days to form a habit." Liza's philosophy is that it takes '33 consecutive days of repeating the same thing over and over – either good or bad- to change and form a new habit. Are you wondering why 33 instead of 21 days? We are creatures of habit and function in a society where everything is measured by "time."

This means we know and understand seconds, minutes, hours, days, weeks, and months. Most days in a month are 31. If we continue a new routine for over 33 consecutive days, then we have done it for over an entire month and are already into the next month. Most think and feel, "If I can do it for over a month, I wonder if I can do this again for the next 33 days," thus placing the new programming into action for the third month.

It is quite simple; instead of coming short in the month (21 days), you have now accomplished something you did not believe was imaginable. While your entire thought process was to do something for 33 days continually, the pressure and the discomfort of "possible failure" is lifted ...and by the second month, the new habit is formed! Bingo! You've succeeded and conquered the old habit. Saying to yourself: "I did it" - "it worked"! Success feeds success!

And what is "it"? IT is YOU.

You have and have had the Power Within all along. For some unknown reason, if this method does not work, we then use hypnosis to find out what other underlying blocks have been lingering within our subconscious mind in need of change. We work to help you feel better, drop negative habits, and begin your new lifestyle of wellness in mind and body. If the intent and the desire are present, then Change is easily achieved!

The hypnosis recording will help you reverse negativity and eliminate your cravings for unwholesome lifestyle behaviors that have created bad habits. As your body begins to balance itself, you will no longer allow yourself to follow physically damaging and mentally straining desires. Use this recording at the end of every day for 33 consecutive days to promote lasting results.

Go to https://healwithin.com/shop to find "Relax and Unwind" along with other helpful audio recordings.

Affirmations for Forgiveness and Resilience

Each day this week, repeat these affirmations:

- I AM now ready to be seen!
- I deserve kindness, compassion, and inner peace.
- Every step I take is a step toward healing and growth.
- I forgive myself for the past and release it with love.
- I am enjoying this process of inner healing.
- I will look sexier. I'm OK with this!
- I appreciate more personal attention.
- I enjoy movement and exercise.
- I AM safe even when attracting attention to myself.
- I can face anything that challenges me.
- I have unlimited energy and motivation.
- I'm proud of myself for doing this!
- No matter the challenge, I will see it through.
- I AM happy being who I am.
- Every positive action I take accelerates my progress.
- I AM ready to allow my body to heal.
- I act purposefully, and things happen.
- I am ready to lovingly *evoke* my past experiences, *embrace* my present situation, and *evolve* to the best version of the new me!
- I can now Stand Up for myself and feel good! YES, I AM.

I Matter!

Your Next Steps: Stay Empowered

Explore More:

- **Workshops and Courses:** Dive deeper into self-discovery and transformation through our tailored workshops.

- **Audio Resources:** Continue reinforcing your journey with any of my empowering hypnosis recordings.

- **Community Support:** Join our community of like-minded individuals who are also embracing their evolution.

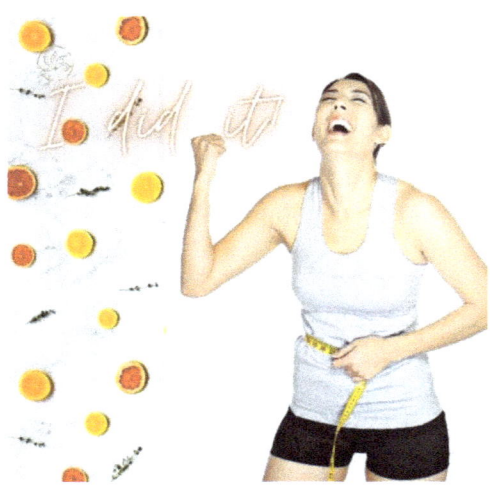

Your Transformational Journey: Celebrating Your Success

Congratulations! You've reached the culmination of your nine-week journey—a milestone worth celebrating. Through commitment, self-reflection, and action, you've equipped yourself with the tools to drop weight, embrace self-love, and stand up for your well-being. Your journey has not only been about weight—it's been about uncovering your strength, honoring your body, and evolving into a more empowered version of yourself. Take a moment to honor your courage and dedication.

Affirmations: The Power of Your Words

Your affirmations have been your guiding light, shaping your thoughts and aligning your actions. Continue with these:

- *I am worthy of love and success.*
- *I only eat when my body is hungry, and I stop when I feel satisfied.*
- *I attract positive energy, and my health improves daily.*
- *I release the past and embrace a brighter future.*

Remember, affirmations are most effective when repeated consistently. Start and end your day with them, integrating them into your routine. Place them in visible spots—your mirror, your car visor, or your desk—and let them remind you of your growth and intentions.

Holistic Health: Your Daily Practices

- Balanced Eating: Eat three balanced meals when hungry, paying attention to portions and nourishing your body. Hydrate by drinking about 64 ounces of water daily.

- Mindful Movement: Incorporate 20-45 minutes of daily activity, whether it's a walk, yoga, or a favorite workout.

- Emotional Awareness: Check in with your feelings. If you're tempted to eat out of stress or boredom, pause and ask yourself what you truly need.

- Self-Reflection: Use your journal to track your thoughts, progress, and insights.

Your imagination is a powerful ally. Use visualization to step into your desired self:

1. Close your eyes and picture yourself at your healthiest, happiest state.

2. Notice how you feel—light, confident, and vibrant.

3. Anchor this image in your mind, repeating affirmations that align with your goals.

Practice self-hypnosis to deepen your connection with your subconscious. Repeat calming affirmations like:
"I am at peace with myself. I welcome harmony and joy into my life."

Your Final Steps

1. Reflect on Your Transformation: What changes do you see and feel? How have you grown emotionally, mentally, and physically?

2. Set New Intentions: What's next for you? Use the tools you've learned to continue your journey of growth.

3. Celebrate Your Success: Treat yourself to something meaningful—a new outfit, a special outing, or a quiet moment of gratitude.

"Our eyes are not only to see; but to project what we witness." ~ Liza

A Message from Liza

You did it. After nine weeks, you've not only completed this program but also laid the foundation for a lifetime of empowerment and self-love. This is just the beginning. Repeat this 33-day journey twice more, and witness your transformation deepen across all levels—mind, body, and spirit.

Remember: *Evoke what was. Embrace what is. Evolve to what will be.* You are a gift. You matter.

For a Seed to Blossom

For a seed to achieve its greatest expression, it must completely come undone.
The shell cracks, its insides come bursting out, and everything begins to change.
To some who do not understand growth, it would look like destruction.
For those who believe, it's just a thought away.

Additional Resources to Support Your Journey

Transforming your relationship with your body and mind doesn't end here. Continue your growth with these resources:

- **_Drop Weight_ Audio Recording**
  This hypnosis recording gently guides your mind to reverse negative thoughts and eliminate cravings for unwholesome food or emotional eating. Your body

begins to balance itself, naturally shifting to healthier patterns without damaging diets.

- *Mind-Body Connection* **Audio Recording**
Designed to accompany you during walks, jogs, or workouts, this recording is infused with specific subliminal messages to motivate you to move your body and embrace a healthier, more active lifestyle.

- **Mala Bracelets**
Use these beautiful bracelets to anchor your affirmations. Rolling your fingers over each bead as you repeat your affirmations helps embed positive changes into your subconscious, strengthening your commitment to your transformation.

I believe in you. Be proud of who you are and allow this process to help you blossom into the best version of yourself. You are creating a healthier, more harmonious relationship with all of YOU—mind, body, and spirit.

"Watch for what unfolds as you blossom." ~ Liza

What Clients Are Saying

"Liza isn't just an expert hypnotherapist. She integrates her work with skill and a passion for helping others." ~ Greg Krikorian, *Business Life Magazine*

"Liza has simply been a blessing for me. Thanks to her expertise, kindness, and talent, I've finally broken free from yo-yo dieting and twisted relationships with food. Liza celebrates your success as much as you do. She's simply terrific, and now I know, 'I Matter.'" ~ Odile Tartaglia

"When I first came to Liza a few years ago, I was over 200 lbs. and miserable. Today, I am at 140 lbs., and my life is fantastic. Liza helped me get past my son's death and instead celebrate his life. I sing your praises. God bless you for helping people." ~ Judith Bennett

A Final Word

You have the tools to create a life of balance, health, and self-love. Remember, this is just the beginning of your journey. Keep revisiting these practices, leaning on the resources provided, and embracing your worth. Please take a moment to share your story or testimonial about how this program has impacted you. Your journey inspires others to believe in themselves and take the first step toward change. As always, I'm here for you, cheering you on with love and gratitude. Lovingly,

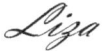

Bonus: Self-Hypnosis Practice for Deeper Healing

Instructions for Self-Hypnosis Practice

All hypnosis is self-hypnosis.
You may read and record this script slowly in your own voice and listen before sleep.
When your own voice speaks with calm and intention, it becomes ten times more nurturing and impactful.
Your subconscious receives it as truth — especially during quiet moments of rest.

After you record it:
Find a quiet, comfortable space where you will not be disturbed.
Sit or recline in a way that feels fully supported.
When ready, gently close your eyes and begin listening to your recording.

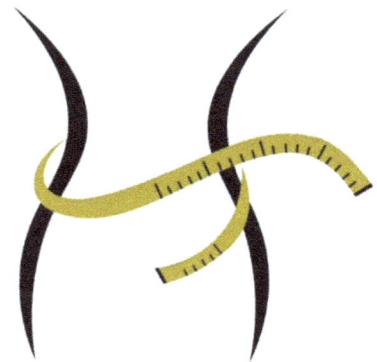

Self-Hypnosis: Drop the Weight

Now that I am fully present with myself...
I invite my body and mind to work together in harmony.
I choose to release the weight I no longer need to carry—
Physically, emotionally, and energetically.

I am ready to accept and appreciate myself just as I am.
I have allowed my body to protect me—even if not consciously.
I can begin to peel away the past hurt.
I can drop all burdens and weight I took upon me.
Today is as good a day as any to forgive myself.
Today I release old patterns and choose a lighter me.

I feel lighter. I feel clearer.
I feel deeply connected to what my body truly needs

Every day, I become more aware of how I nourish myself—
Not just with food, but with thoughts, movement, rest, and self-love.

I choose healthier.
I leave or give the last bite away.
I can feel lighter.
I am safe.

I speak kindly to my body.
I listen when it whispers, and I honor when it speaks.
The more I drop the weight that never belonged to me,
The more I rise in my worth, power, and presence.

My body is wise.
My body is strong.
My body is healing.

I trust the process.

When I am ready, I take a deep breath in...
I bring gentle movement back to my fingers and toes...
And I return to full awareness—lighter, freer, and filled with gratitude for myself.

About Liza

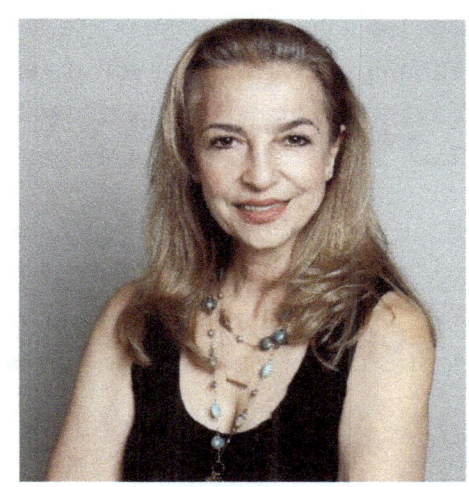

As a Certified Clinical Hypnotherapist, Liza Boubari is one of the most reputable specialists in emotional weight and wellness in the Greater Los Angeles area. With over two decades of experience, Liza has helped countless individuals heal within and transform their relationships with their bodies and emotions.

"Life changed for me when I learned to connect my mind and body, shedding not just physical weight but the emotional burdens that held me back." Liza's journey of overcoming her own challenges with weight, self-worth, and health through hypnotherapy and self-awareness fuels her mission to help others reclaim their lives. Through *Stand Up to Slim Down*, Liza combines guided imagery, empowering affirmations, and intentional insights to support readers in breaking free from emotional eating, self-doubt, and unhealthy habits.

Her professional expertise and compassionate approach have empowered countless individuals to heal emotional wounds, release limiting beliefs, and embrace healthier, more fulfilling lives with confidence and clarity.

The work you have done is a testament to your courage and commitment. Trust that you are exactly where you need to be, guided by a higher energy that has always been within you. Take the first step toward healing within—you're worth it.

Book your session today. I encourage you to get the _Drop Weight_ and _Mind-Body Connection_ (move your body) self-hypnosis audio to reinforce your journey. Visit **HealWithin.com** for resources, tools, and more inspirational success stories.

Our Mission:

To empower individuals to heal within by uncovering and transforming layers of hurt and pain buried deep in the unconscious mind.
Evoke - Embrace - Evolve – You Matter

If you or someone you know is ready to begin the journey of healing mind and body, reach out for a free, no-obligation consultation. Take the first step toward creating a healthier, happier you. Let's start your journey of healing today.

Contact Us:

 818-551-1501

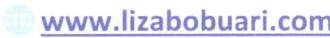 www.lizabobuari.com

www.healwithin.com